Fundamentals in Management of Bronchial Asthma

Fundamentals in Management of Bronchial Asthma

Hamid Yahay Hussain

ELIVA PRESS

ISBN: 978-99949-8-083-3

Cover Design: Eliva Press
Cover Image: Freepik Premium
Email: info@elivapress.com
Website: www.elivapress.com

This Eliva Press imprint is published by the registered company Eliva Press Global Ltd. part of Eliva Press S.R.L. Publishing Group

The registered company address is: Pope Hennessy Street Level 2, Hennessy Tower Port Louis, Mauritius
Eliva Press S.R.L. Publishing Group address is: Bulevardul Moscova 21, Chisinau, Moldova, Europe

Fundamentals in Asthma management

Dr. Hamid Yahya Hussain,

Consultant physician

Table of contents

Title Page

Abstract

Chronic respiratory diseases are among the leading causes of global chronic diseases mortality. WHO has estimated that worldwide, around 300 million people have asthma, (WHO, 2009). Bronchial asthma is the most prevalent chronic disease among children right now (WHO, 2010) it is still a public health concern for all countries, regardless of the level of income or development (Myers T, Kelley CF et al, 2005). Despite effective treatment, asthma is associated with high morbidity and significant mortality so far (Higgins PS, Wakefield D, Cloutier MM, 2005). Yet, with high prevalence of asthma , it is better to mention that significant reduction in asthma mortality has been achieved due to better asthma management procedures as well as good educational programs applied worldwide, but asthma management still encountering real challenges among certain targets like elderly due to poor recognition and under treatment due to failure of perceive problem and difficulties in use therapy, teenager groups and low socio economical classes always have multiple triggers and poor compliance with the drug.

Introduction, Asthma, true burden

In the late 20th century, we witnessed enormous progress in the epidemiology of asthma and allergic diseases. .(Liebhart J, Malolepszy J, Wojtyniak B, Pisiewicz K, Plusa K, Gladysz U.2007) 'The highest deaths burden of the disease affects the low- and lower-middle income countries. About (255 000) people died of asthma in 2005 worldwide, placing an enormous strain on health resources in many countries, and is a major cause of hospitalization for chronic diseases in children in western world. In the United States of America, 15 million people have asthma, and of them, nearly 4.8 million are children (Al-Thamiri D, Al-Kutaisi W, 2005), it was estimated that asthma costs around 13.8 billion dollars for the year 2000 in United States. In UAE Often, asthma is under-diagnosed and under-treated, leading to reduce quality of life for the patients, and increases the burden on their families (Ministry of health UAE, 2008).

Asthma extensively strains the health systems, where in USA more than 10 million of health care visits are done by asthmatic patients and around half a million people requires hospital admissions to manage their asthma annually (Al-Ghamdi BR et al ,2008). In the Middle East region, asthma continues to be of public health concern, AIRGEN survey 2009 was conducted in 5 countries in the Middle East countries including UAE, OMAN, JORDAN, LEBANON and Kuwait showed that 23% of patient had been hospitalized due to asthma and 52% visited emergency room in the past year (Khadadah, M. Mahboub, B, 2009). The prevalence of Asthma in Saudi Arabia is as high as 12% in general population and 23% among school children. These figures are comparable to the prevalence figures in UAE, where the prevalence of asthma is 12% in the general population and 13% among the school children. In 2007, the total number of visits to the primary health care centers in UAE due to asthma was 36,498 with a rate of 12.19 visits per 1,000 populations. The prevalence of childhood asthma has been reported to vary (1%–30%) in different populations. These variations are possibly due to differing exposures to respiratory infections, indoor or outdoor pollution and diet. (UAE/MOH.2009)

In the United Arab Emirates the prevalence of asthma diagnosed by physicians among governmental primary school children was 13% in addition the wheeze by history was 15.6%. There were 57 deaths (from a total of 6002 deaths that) due to asthma and bronchitis in 2003 which mean that this diseases specific death rate is 1.41 per 100,000. (Alsuwaidi S .2009).Hence it is important to implement primary prevention measures and identify cost-effective interventions to control asthma, such as surveillance, appropriate asthma treatment and management. (Al Thamiri D, 2005)

Primary health care area is the frontline of encountering asthma cases in terms of diagnosis and treatment event when asthma presented as an emergency (lyte et al, 2007, Scullion, 2005).

As a primary health care physician whose entitled to run out services , including management of asthma at school level which is quite exciting and challenging issue for me so far , as to the high prevalence among students and relatively week capacity of asthma management infrastructure at schools. A greater awareness of asthma in schools and health checks for teenagers in general practice may help to improve diagnosis, and strategies to discourage cigarette smoking should be targeted at young people with asthma (john F Price, 2010). According to the asthma management guidelines and local national school health guideline available currently in Dubai, patient has the right to have access to the trained staff and professional code of conduct to ensure receiving as optimum management as he needs (BTS/SIGN, 2007). enrolled with Asthma management, through which a case study approach(methodology) will be adopted to reflect the orientation level to the course content, this work is going to examine the assessment and management of an adolescent patient who will be called (Rashid) for the sake of confidentiality, he

Human airways facts, functions and structures:

Rashid presenting symptoms are mainly chronic and intermittent attacks of dry cough, tightness of the chest, breathlessness and wheezes. As Asthma is a chronic inflammatory disease, with episodic occurrences of airflow obstruction, hypersensitivity and responsiveness to various stimuli, which lead to breathlessness, wheezing, coughing and tightness of the chest which is resolving spontaneously or by treatment (Gina, 2006. BTS/Sign, 2007), inflammation considered to be the main underlying pathogenesis through two main mechanisms, bronchial hyper responsiveness and airway restriction (Colgate and Douglass, 2006). The main function of the human airways system is to deliver oxygen and remover carbon dioxide from the body and, maintain blood PH.

Respiratory system in mankind consist of upper and lower one, as for upper, it is composes of nose, Para nasal sinuses, pharynx and larynx which has number of important functions like smell, humidification of air, taste and speech while for the lower one it compose of trachea, bronchi, bronchioles and alveoli, the principle function of this part is gas exchange ($O2$, $co2$) between the air and circulation. Lung is highly vascular organ enriched with blood vessels and controlled by Central nervous system. Walls conducting airway are characterized by Mucous membrane lining, muscular or cartilaginous layer and connective tissue out layer (Murray JF, 1994).

Asthma is classified physiologically as a variable obstruction to air flow, and pathologically with overdeveloped mucus glands, airway thickening due to scarring and inflammation, and bronco constriction. Bronchial inflammation also causes narrowing due to edema and swelling caused by an immune response to allergens. (Nunn JF, 1994).

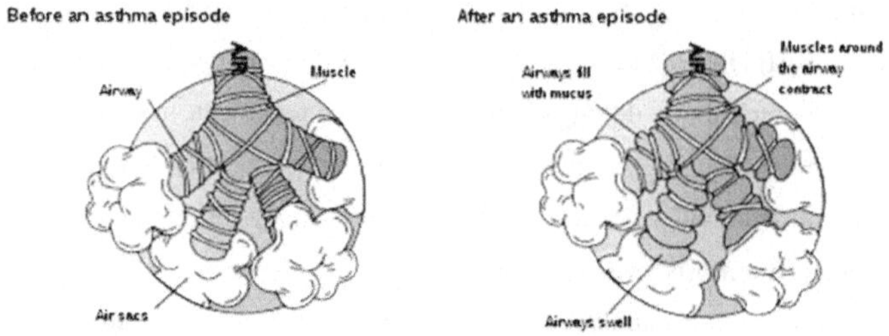

During an asthma episode, inflamed airways react to environmental triggers such as smoke, dust, or pollen or others. The airways narrow and produce excess mucus, making it difficult to breathe. In essence, asthma is the result of an immune response in the bronchial airways (Murray JF, 1994).

The airways of asthma patients are "hypersensitive" to certain triggers, also known as stimuli). (It is usually classified as type I hypersensitivity.) In response to exposure to these triggers, the bronchi (large airways) contract into spasm (an "asthma attack"). Inflammation soon follows, leading to a further narrowing of the airways and excessive mucus production, which leads to coughing and other breathing difficulties as in Rashid case. Broncho spasm may resolve spontaneously in 1–2 hours, or in about 50% of subjects, may become part of a 'late' response, where this initial insult is followed 3–12 hours later with further broncho constriction and inflammation (Martini F, 2006)

Bronchial inflammation:

It was identified that this patient (Rashid) had developed frequent rhinitis symptoms between March and June for almost 4-5 days a week with itching , runny nose , sneezing and watery eyes for which he was put on anti-allergic agents, The mechanisms behind allergic asthma—i.e., asthma resulting from an immune response to inhaled allergens—are the best understood of the causal factors. In both people with asthma and people who are free of the disease, inhaled allergens that find their way to the inner airways are ingested by a type of cell known as antigen-presenting cells, or APCs. APCs then "present" pieces of the allergen to other immune system cells. In most people, these other immune cells

(T_H0 cells) "check" and usually ignore the allergen molecules. In asthma patients, however, these cells transform into a different type of cell (T_H2), for reasons that

The "hygiene hypothesis" postulates that an imbalance in the regulation of these T_H cell types in early life leads to a long-term domination of the cells involved in allergic responses over those involved in fighting infection. The suggestion is that for a child being exposed to microbes early in life, taking fewer antibiotics, living in a large family, and growing up in the country stimulate the T_H1 response and reduce the odds of developing asthma. (Llli S, 2001).

Pathogenesis

The fundamental problem in asthma appears to be immunological: young children in the early stages of asthma show signs of excessive inflammation in their airways. Epidemiological findings give clues as to the pathogenesis: the incidence of asthma seems to be increasing worldwide, and asthma is now very much common in affluent countries.

In 1968, Andor Szentivanyi first described The Beta Adrenergic Theory of Asthma; in which blockage of the Beta-2 receptors of pulmonary smooth muscle cells causes asthma. Szentivanyi' s Beta Adrenergic Theory is a citation classic using the Science Citation Index and has been cited more times than any other article in the history of the Journal of Allergy and Clinical Immunology.In 1995 Szentivanyi and colleagues demonstrated that IgE blocks beta-2 receptors. Since overproduction of IgE is central to all a topic diseases, this was a watershed moment in the world of allergy

What factors should we figure out in asthma? :

It has been recognized also that Rashid Constant symptoms which presented for long time is in favors of continuous exposure to environmental triggers, predisposing factors. The risk of developing asthma is a combination of two factors: genetic predisposition and environmental exposure to allergens. Indoor allergens (e.g. dust mites), outdoor allergens (e.g. pollens), tobacco smoke, and air pollution can trigger asthma attacks.(Kumar P, Clark M (Ed.). 1998)Other triggering factors include cold air, physical exercise, extreme emotions and certain medications, such as aspirin, non-steroidal anti-inflammatory drugs and beta-blockers

The rate of asthma increases as communities adopt western lifestyles and become urbanised. With the projected increase in the proportion of the world's population that is urban from 45% to 59% in 2025, there is likely to be a marked increase in the number of asthmatics worldwide over the next two decades. It is estimated that there may be an additional 100 million persons with asthma by 2025 Kudzyte J, Geisha E, Bojarskas J the prevalence of asthma in different countries varies from 1.2% to 32.2% and depends on age, sex, race, and place of living. Prevalence of asthma is increasing, with concomitant increases in morbidity, economic costs, and in some countries, mortality. It has a significant impact on the quality of life. Exposure of an allergic individual to the below allergen results in the development of early asthma and late asthma response:

- Indoor allergens
- Outdoor allergens
- Food triggers
- Indoor air pollution
- Medications
- Exercise
- Concurrent medical conditions (infections e.g., viral upper respiratory infection, bronchitis, sinusitis, allergic rhinitis,
- gastro esophageal reflux disease)
- Psychological stress
- Occupational asthma

Rashid medical and family history was strongly associated with exposure to a number of asthma predisposing factors, he has got a positive history of sever a topic dermatitis during his childhood period, his father and one of his older brothers were asthmatics individuals , allergic rhinitis was about to be confirmed recently with Rashid case. Studies showed that asthma incidence affected by socio-economic status, environmental hygienic circumstance, life style factors, occupational exposure, body weight and physical activity efforts.

Early exposure to sensitizing materials e.g. tobacco, house dust mites and domestic pets significantly associated with childhood asthma, (Illi S, 2006), and this is in fact present In Rashid case as he was exposed to passive smoking since his father was smoker. It has been suggested as well that early exposure to antibiotics may be correlated with asthma precipitation especially with misdiagnosis of respiratory tract infection as most of the infections are viral. More hygienic theory went far beyond as hygienic status will defiantly lead to decrease the opportunity of exposure to Microorganisms and decrease the opportunity of immunological challenges where developing of powerful immune system stay beyond, as asthma pathogenesis is mainly related to immune system , and weak immune system is significantly associated with asthma incidence .

As for older age group, smoking weather active or passive stay the main trigger behind asthma attaches as well as exposure to different occupational substance at workplace which may reach up to 25% of the diseases among adults. (Hoskins G et al(2000).Asthma can be precipitated by drug as well , aspirin and non-steroidal anti-inflammatory medicines are the main groups of drugs attributed to asthma , stress and emotional reaction are distinctly triggering asthmatic patients and greatly correlated with developing of asthma attach . (Platt-Mills, TEA.2005), Asthma can lead to acute and chronic complications like a telecast secondary to mucus plugging, pneumothorax, mediastinal emphysema, chest deformity and growth disturbance and irreversibility.

Comprehensive Assessment of asthma

Asthma diagnosis is a multi approaches process including elaborated patient's history accompanied with pulmonary function assessment, adding to these the clinical presentation of the patient as reflected by signs and symptoms which may or may not be present at the time of diagnoses, putting in the consideration the severity and the duration of signs and symptoms. The extent of functional and structural limitation of the airflow is in fact the main determinant for the severity of the disease and the status of reversibility of the damages, patient centered approach is an effective one through acknowledging symptoms impact on daily life activities (BTS/SIGN, 2007.GINA, 2006) and by using the three keys questions (appendix 5) which indicate poor control in case of positive answer. Response to treatment is very suggestive about the diagnosis and the presence of environmental trigger factors. From the chronic nature, the frequent exacerbation attacks and poor school performance of Rashid case, a question has been raised by myself weather or not Rashid has gone through proper assessment procedures and identified the exact description of his status in terms of quantitative and qualitative assessment.

Revising Rashid medical file, taking full history and using structured assessment approach (Holgate and Douglass,2006)(Levy et al,2006) by interview and carrying out some physiological laboratory investigations showed that multiple prescriptions has been issued for Rashid by different doctors, reflecting a fact that this patient is kept turning over many doctors seeking more help and get less benefits which kept him suffering and happen to affect his daily activities and commitments in the school as well as the absence of precautionary measures due to lack of education and awareness. Asthmatic attacks precipitated frequently and even at rest status recently, and responded partially to short acting B2 agonist inhaler, which all in favor uncontrolled asthma. As one interview is not enough to make assessment, I planed with Rashid and his family to have more assessment interviews according to his earliest convenience.

Rashid has passive smoking history as his father was smoker, they have kept pets in their house and frequently on antibiotics by different physicians on different chest attacks, and on his way to school he has to pass a heavily polluted area of factories.

It was noticed by the class supervisor that Rashid academic performance was clearly declining and sickness absences were noticeably reported across the last three months .School nurse and school doctor reported frequent asthma manifestations which are strongly suggestive of his school dropout and uncontrolled status of asthma (Levy et al , 2006).

Physical examination carried out for Rashid revealed, continuous wheezing, rapid respiratory rate and pulse rate and continuous dry cough, and that were increased significantly in the late weeks. Rashid PEFR shows significant reduction, more than 25% measure in liter per minute and showed that his PEFR finding as it is valid method of diagnosis (Booker ,2007) (Gina , 2006) indicated that the value was less than 70% of total volume of air exhaled during the first second of breathing (FEV1/FVC)ratio which should be at least 80% or above of expected to be considered as a normal

While normal spirometry can expected among asthmatic patient especially during their wellbeing periods.

Rashid best PEFR was (410) L/Min, representing about 65% of the expected value of 656 l/Min according to his age, sex and height (Asthma UK, 2007b). More ,two weeks Peak flow diary was recommended to Rashid case twice daily in advance to asthma medication, according to (Gina,2006,BTS/Sign,2007) a reduction of about 20% and above at least 60 l/Min for three day a week for two week is a diagnostic test for asthma and a diurnal variation between morning and evening of about 10% and more is considered to be abnormal, and that was quite positive in this patient . Rashid has been taught how to use the apparatus and how to recording the reading accordingly and trained properly on the maneuver of using Peak flue diary (asthma UK, 2004) as it is ideal to record PEF on a daily base in asthmatic patients. Reversibility testing, steroid reversibility testing and exercise testing were all done for my patient and were all suggestive of asthma diagnosis, Immunoglobulin E (IGE) Radio immune specific allergen test, skin prick test and radiological assessment were carried out as part of comprehensive asthma assessment where all gave good evidences in Rashid case .

So far, I have to exclude other possible of chronic obstructive pulmonary diseases, Upper respiratory airway obstruction, vocal cord dysfunction, cystic fibrosis, pulmonary edema, hyperventilation, viral associated wheezes and allergic bronco-pulmonary aspergellosis for which necessary investigation and examinations were carries out.

Asthma pharmacology:

The main pharmacological strategies in asthma are bronchodilator and anti-inflammatory agents separated or in compensation in different dosage and adjustment according to the case assessment, thus Rashid was given Short acting B2 agonist as required plus corticosteroid as inhalation 500 mcg/day to be used 2-3 times via pressurized –metered dose inhaler (PMDI) on acute status

I was surprised that so far Rashid did not exposed to training or demonstration how to use his inhaler and what is the right technique which in fact contributed to his uncontrolled status of asthma, when Rashid asked to demonstrate using inhaler properly, it was totally incorrect technique. (Thomas et al, 2007) refer to a fact that majority of asthmatic patient were using inhaler techniques improperly. Following the standard of using inhaler technique criteria (Burn,2008) as well as asthma UK website(asthma UK,2006) Rashid was not able to do inhaler technique correctly which was part of his uncontrolled status

. Socio cultural, economic, environmental and educational background of Rashid family contributed to the large extent in making him UN controlled case of asthma.

In fact diagnosis of asthma in adolescent age is particularly difficult (thorax, 1996) as there is always reluctance issue, usually separate individuals from their peers and compliance with the therapy is not good as there is un- willingness to undertake regular therapy. Death rate is almost four times higher in comparison with younger age group. Management always required different approaches with multidisciplinary plan to encourage communications. Psychological problem can be commonly found in this age like vocal cord dysfunction, always social and psychological history has to be noticed when control prove to be difficult as these factors has an important bearing on diagnosis and management.

I extremely believe in Patient centered consultation as aiming to explore patient understanding of the problem and intervention such as pharmacological (Fradd, 1996), and enabling the patient to negotiate and contribute to the plan of care, this approach include provision of the patient with necessary information and sort out his concerns as was followed in current case . Health education and asthma education are decisive strategy in asthma management outcomes (Gleeson C, 1998) for which reason it was greatly utilized in management of Rashid case.

Multi-disciplinary team is another competent strategy in asthma management , effort of medical social worker, community psychiatric nurse, occupational therapist, pharmacist, lab technicians , nurse and physician are all have their own roles in asthma management and contribute effectively in asthma management outcome (Keely D.1993) which was clearly considered though out handling of this case. revising medical history ,drug history, socio-educational status of the family were all of significance in relation to the outcome, neither the patient nor his family were aware enough about the diseases and precipitating factor, parents were busy with different commitments and there was clear absent of family role and care system.

As a conclusion , Rashid asthma can be described as an uncontrolled one, sever and threatening for his daily activities due to bad pharmacological regime, poor education ,lack of training about inhaler techniques , low awareness about precipitating and triggering factors, absence of action plan and support from family due to their overwhelmed commitments . Other diffential diagnoses have been raised and sort out as asthma presenting symptoms can be similar to other respiratory tract disorders.

In the light of the abovementioned fact, I decide to adopt multi level asthma management strategy for Rashid to remove all contributors to his bad management status. Symptom based, and Peak flow dairy based policy explained to Rashid through demonstration sessions and providing educational materials, his parents we approached in aim to enrolling them effectively in the asthma management plan, training the patient on proper utilization of inhaler techniques and guideline to avoiding triggering conditions, close teachers role was identified and discussed at school . And an effective pharmacological plan was adopted as following:

Adding to the previous abovementioned medicine a long acting inhaled B2 agonist was proposed ,Rashid was followed up for two weeks on the new regime and assessed thoroughly after , he showed lots of benefits , yet control status still in adequate which indicate to increase inhaled steroid dose to 800Mcg/ day, (Gina,2008), were the symptoms controlled so far , I put Rashid on two weeks assessment and follow up schedule after improving and discussed with his family the possibility of adding Leucocratic receptor antagonist or SR theophyline as a part of asthma step up management strategy if indicated , comprehensive evaluation for the management plan in terms of spirometry findings and PEFR as well as clinical assessment and daily life activities . Diurnal PEFR variability was in favor of Asthma diagnosis, clinically asthma can be presented in different form , it can be presented as mild persistent for more than once a week and less than daily with variability of 22-26% of PEFR more than 60 L/Min(Gina, 2008). Rashid went through comprehensive educational program focusing on concerning treatment and how to control underlying path physiology and minimizing symptoms and optimizing lung function (BTS/SIGN,2007) Holgate,2007).

Management strategies of asthma:

Step wising approach in Rashid treatment was highlighted to him and his family, according to the Gina Guideline five pharmacological alternatives steps has been proved in management of asthma (As shown in the appendix 1) based on asthma control level with the concept of stepping up treatment and stepping down as the symptoms increased or decreased to achieve best control . Rashid treatment was within step three of Gina guideline, to be monitored whether he needs to step up to level four or down to level two or stay at current level.) As one of effective measure taken with Rashid in aiming to improve his emotional and social image , he has been advised to participate in class sports activities with a precaution of giving Short acting B2 agonist 10 mints before exercising to relief the symptoms .

As the main path physiology of asthma is the inflammation process and its squeal , corticosteroid agent stay the most effective option available so far in asthma management (Holgate and Doglas,2006) with different inflammatory characteristics (zdanwicz,2007). The evidences showed that almost three quarters of all asthmatic patients can achieve good control through steroid treatment option (Guiard et al, 2006). As for the prolog untreated inflammation possibility of airway re modeling is quite true, for which treatment with steroid in such patient should be continued for long time even when the symptoms controlled. (Roberts, 2002)

Inhaler corticosteroid has no side effect in general except of some local side effect like mouth Candidiasis and some dysphonic changes which is in fact can be reduces significantly if spacer techniques used for the patient , on the other side systematic treatment with corticosteroid has many side effects , some of which are even serious like cushion disease and demineralization of bone (Holtage and Douglass ,2006), as for the acute symptom , it is better to mention that Inhaler corticosteroid is of no benefit to relief the symptom , for that any patient has to carry a short acting (B2)agonist agent in case of acute exacerbation of signs and symptoms . Rashid has been through full discussions about the airway inflammation and the role of ICS in relieving the symptom within a month where Rashid can be engaged actively in exercises without any symptom. As Rashid showed lack of adherence to the treatment in the previous period so assuring him about the benefit of ICS, side effect and its vital role in asthma management (Newell, 2006), Some literature from Gina guideline for asthma management as supportive evidences were given to Rashid. B2 agonist agent was highlighted as well , its effect , the way it affect smooth muscle and stimulating muscle relaxation which last from 3-5 hours (Jordan and White,2001) and the main side effects lie palpitation , tachycardia and tremors and the importance of adjustment between CS and B2agonist agent . Inhaler technique is one of the cornerstones in asthma management as good inhalation mean symptoms free and control, inspire of being using inhaler since long time Rashid did not meet the inhalation technique effectively so far, demonstrating was done in front of him and demonstration by the patient then done. Rashid has been told that to minimize local side effect of corticosteroid , spacer technique can be utilized through which particle size can be reduced and increase airway deposition (Thomas et al ,2007) , yet Rashid was un enthusiastic to use spacer, following inhaler technique assessment , Rashid advised to keep carrying his inhaler all the time as he showed frequent forgotten to use it . All treatment process has been assessed, adherence to medication , proper inhaler techniques , patient plan and patient education, asthma control parameter was reflect by Rashid PEFR improvement to be exceeding 580 l /min and his PEFR diary showed very minimum variation(Batman et al,2004). He reported no night time or day time symptoms and using SABA twice a week before exercising and enrolled in heavy exercises without developing symptoms which all in favor of good asthma control (Steven et al, 2002). So far Rashid is coping with normal daily life activities and the plan to keep on this regime for the next three month.

Acute exacerbation of asthma has no relation to asthma severity (partridge et al,2006) , this is as well applicable even for the controlled patients who are borne to develop at least 6 attaches per year ,this raise the question of discussing the issue of triggering factor with patient and families and developing a plan of triggers avoidance , yet avoidance is not an easy process, it may require a routine allergens testing program ,based on this a n extensive pragmatic program was considered for Rashid case to be able to targeting his triggers which are not easy to be avoided like exercises, pollens , viruses, since exercises are essential for healthy life Rashid was encouraged to participate conditional to be adherent to the Asthma management guideline by using SABA. Clear massages were given to Rashid about the warming up slowly and avoid cold air. The pollen in case of Rashid asthma still challenging issue as he got Rhinitis and rhinitis associate with 50% risk of hospitalization by asthma exacerbation(Thomas, 2006). More cut grass outdoor is quite common and it is not practical to be indoor to avoid exposure, antihistamine is no longer effective , I put Rashid on intranasal steroid spray as treatment of rhinitis which is save and adequate . as for viral infection it is still challenging in asthma management since it is deteriorating the asthma , I advise Rashid to avoid any risky situation and if develop any vial like illnesses he has to attend physicians and step up of the treatment at earlier stages , more I put Rashid on annual influenza vaccine as effective preventive strategy .

The Inspire study, 2006 showed that there is window period that last about 5 days by which patients confronting early signs and symptoms of deterioration that keep worsening until the attack this mechanism has been thoroughly explained to Rashid and his family stressed on to increase medication to avoid attack. As studies revealed the significant benefit of developing asthma management plan on the severity and frequency, self-monitoring plan was established to Rashid (Jarvis,2006) including , symptom monitoring , PEFR and reviewing regular medication under my supervision, Rashid was quite happy and enthusiastic to have part of action in asthma management plan (Gibson et al,2002). Rashid was willing to contribute in treatment decision making in spite of some study showed that some patient do want to play passive role (Caress et al ,2005), there was off course some hesitation to have an active role at the starting , this changed dramatically to positive and active role with proceeding in understanding , knowledge enhancement and skills upgrading .

Check list was developed for Rashid for worsening symptoms that have significant medication review, in relation to increasing night time or day time symptom and increasing reliever usage (Roberts, 2002), I told Rashid that upon consistency of asthma control process we are going to skipped him from PEFR diary (Buist,2006) reveled that symptom monitoring is as effective as PEFR diary Yet if symptom increase Rashid can be back to PEFR diary as 80% Reading considered to be normal, Urgent medical help and triggers were also discussed with the patient including decrease the effectiveness of reliever and increasing symptoms, difficulty of speaking due to breathlessness, Asthma attack card and asthma leaflets were provided for reinforcement of his information .

Two months before Rhinitis season , I planned to review Rashid status and his protocol through which I will stress on adherence to the medication, self-management advises , inhaler technique assessment, nasal spray technique and identify any potentials in term of control to an at risk period. It was revealed by Goal study ,2004 ,that the patient without stepped down treatment for the last 6 months they showed less exacerbation, better lung function test and better life quality while poor control is still the main indicator for stepping up of the treatment, Rashid needs another assessment after that season in a frequency of once a year to look to asthma control, quality of life and as regular contact strategy in asthma management is significantly better than asthma crisis management on the eventual outcome as shown by living and Breathing study, 2004.

Conclusion:

It was concluded that in asthma management there are many pitfalls that can hamper the required outcome which are identified at multiple levels starting from understanding of asthma process by the patient and what triggering them, what avoidance procedures can be followed, asthma assessment both by physician and patient himself is still quite challenging and the proper management according to the different levels by asthma management guideline and how to keep maintaining long term control , patient and family education element and inhaler techniques are quite practical problems that lead to asthma management failure frequently .

Rashid was extremely challenging case for me ,he went through different physicians consultations and he has in fact different levels of obstacles against asthma management success, this patient was about to lose his social life and productivity as well as the health threatens issues , I can finally say that Asthma management is an art and science approach, it fulfils good knowledge and skills as well as developing a standard practice and the whole process has to be patient centralized process, as family physician I come across hundreds of bad management of asthma and malpractice which cost the patient and the health care system quite high , I deeply think that focusing on standardization of the asthma management and training of the health care provider to be on the truck is the key area. .

Annexes:

Appendix (1) Stepwise management in Adult

Step5: Continuous or frequent use of Oral steroid Use daily steroid tablet in lowest dose provide good control. Maintain high dose inhaled steroid 2000Mic/day Consider other treatment to minimize the use of steroid tablets Refer patient to the special care
Step4: persistent poor control Consider trial of Increasing inhaled steroid up to 2000mic/ day Addition of fourth drug e.g. lukotirene receptor antagonists theophyline, B2 agonist tablet.
Step3: Add On Therapy 1. add inhaled long acting B2 agonist(LABA) 2. Assess control of asthma Good response to LABA continue to LABA Benefit from LABA but the control still inadequate continues LABA and increase inhaled dose of steroid to 800Mic/day in not already on this dose. No benefit of LABA stop it and continue with inhaled steroid to 800mic/day if control still in adequate institute trial of other therapies e.g. Leukotriene receptor antagonist or SR theophyline.
Step2: Regular preventer therapy Add inhaled steroid of 200-800 Mic/ day 400 mic is an appropriate starting dose for many patients Start at dose of inhaled steroid appropriate to the severity
Step1: Mild intermittent asthma Inhaled B2 agonist as required

Appendix (2) Asthma management / Long term objectives

3. As minimum as possible signs and symptom day and night times
4. Least possible need for reliever medication
5. Free limits of physical activities
6. Normal physiological lung function test.
7. Minimum or no medication side effect
8. prevent asthma mortality

BTS/SIGN (2007), GINA, (2006).

Appendix (3) Proper inhaler technique BMDI

1. pre use shaking of the inhaler
2. Cap removal
3. Exhale in a gentle
4. Fit the mouth piece in a mouth prior to inhalation
5. By starting of inhalation process, depress the canister to release a dose of medication.
6. Breathe in for the maximum capacity of breathing and hold the breath for 10 second in.
7. second dose can be taken after one minute

Burns D (2008)

Appendix (4) Peak expiratory flow record.

1. Start with zero pointing on the Meter.
2. Sit upright or stand.
3. Hold the meter horizontally with open hole for air exhale
4. Take maximum breath in
5. Place the mouth piece between the teeth in order not to be occluded by the tong.
6. Blow Down the meter as hard as possible.
7. There should be no any delay between breath in and blow down the meter.
8. Blow out with sharp and short huff.
9. Read the pointer
10. Take time for recover and repeat the test at least twice time more.
11. The three reading should be the 20 l/min of each other
12. Record the highest reading.

Booker R (2007)

Appendix (5) Three Key Questions for asthma control

In the last week/month

1. Have you hade difficulty in sleeping because of your asthma symptoms (including cough)? Yes/no
2. Have you had your usual asthma symptom during the day (Cough, Wheze, chest tightness or breathlessness)? Yes? No
3. 3. Has your asthma interfered with your usual activities (e.g., housework, work, school etc?).

Scullion GE (2005b)

Appendix (6) the control of asthma is defined as:

1. No day time symptoms.
2. No night time awaking due to asthma.
3. No need for rescue medications.
4. No exacerbation
5. No limitation on activity including exercise.
6. Normal lung function with minimal side effects.

(BTS, 2008).

Appendix 7 Composite measure of asthma control-the gaining optimal asthma control (GOAL) study:

1. Have you had any day time asthma?
2. Have you had to use blue inhaler much lately?
3. Dose your asthma wake up you at night?
4. Do you ever avoid doing things because of your asthma?
5. Have you had to make an emergency visit recently because of your asthma?
6. Have you had any treatment related side effects resulting in treatment change?
7. Has your morning PEF been less than 80% predicted

(Batman et al, 2004)

References:

Al-Ghamdi BR, Mahfouz AA, Abdelmoneim I, Khan MY, Daffallah AA. Altitude and bronchial asthma in south-western Saudi Arabia. Eastern Mediterranean Health Journal. 2008; 1(14): 17-23.

Al-Thamiri D, Al-Kubaisy W, Ali SH. Asthma prevalence and severity among primary-school children in Baghdad. Eastern Mediterranean Health Journal. 2005; ½(11): 79-86.

Alsuwaidi S, Abdulla A, Bernsen R. Prevalence and risk factors of asthma among adolescents and their parents in Al-Ain (United Arab Emirates). Respiration. 2009; doi: 10.1159/000219248

Asthma in United Arab Emirates. Ministry of Health (MOH). Accessed October 26th, 2009. Available from: http://www.moh.gov.ae/en/Page_573.aspx

Asthma. World Health Organization (WHO). Accessed October 26th, 2009, available from http://www.who.int/topics/asthma/en/.

Asthma. World Health Organization (WHO). Accessed May 26th, 2010, available from http://www.who.int/topics/asthma/en/

Asthma UK (2007b) Emergency asthma care CD-ROM version 2.

Asthma UK (2007c) asthma medication card .available from info@asthma.org.uk

Asthma UK (2006) Demo to help your patient with their inhaler technique @ www.asthma.org.uk/how we help/publishing _ reports/index.html(last access on 11/6/2010).

Asthma UK (2005) personal asthma action plan .available from info@asthma.org.uk

Asthma UK 2004 your peak flow diary. Available at info@ asthma.org.uk.

Alsuwaidi S, Abdulla A, Bernsen R. Prevalence and risk factors of asthma among adolescents and their parents in Al-Ain (United Arab Emirates). Respiration. 2009; doi: 10.1159/000219248.

Al-Thamiri D, Al-Kubaisy W, Ali SH. Asthma prevalence and severity among primary-school children in Baghdad. Eastern Mediterranean Health Journal. 2005; ½(11): 79-86.

Bateman ED, Boushey HA, Bousquet J (2004). Can guideline-defined asthma control be achieved/the gaining optimal Asthma control study/?. American journal of respiratory and critical care medicine.170, 8,836-844.

Bener A, Abdulrazzaq YM, Debuse P, Al-Mutawwa J. Prevalence of asthma among Emirates school children. European J of Epidemiology. 1994; 10: 271-273.

Booker R (2007) Peak expiratory flow measurement. Nursing standard.21, 39, 42-43.

British thoracic society, Scottish intercollegiate guideline network (BTS/SIGN, 2007) British guideline on management of asthma. a national clinical guideline, revised edition BTS/SIGN, 2007 edinbburgh.http://www.sign.ac.uk/guidelines/fultex/63/index.html.(last accessed (2/5/2010).

British thoracic society, Scottish intercollegiate guideline network (BTS/SIGN, 2007) British guideline on management of asthma. A national clinical guideline, revised edition BTS/SIGN, 2007 edinbburgh.http://www.sign.ac.uk/guidelines/fultex/63/index.html.(last accessed (11/5/2010).

Buist As, Vollmer WM, Wilson SR et al (2006). A randomized clinical trial of peak flow versus symptom monitoring in older adults with asthma. American journal of respiratory and critical care medicine.174, 1077-1087.

Burn D (2007) Management of patients with asthma and allergic rhinitis. Nursing standards 21, 26, 48-56.

Burns D (2008) practical aspects of asthma management. Practice nurse.35, 4, 23-27

.. Preventing chronic diseases a vital investment. World Health Organization (WHO). 2005.

Caress AL,Beaver K, Luker K et al (2005) Involvements in treatment decisions : what do adults with asthma wants and what do they gets, results of cross sectional survey . Thorax.60:199-205.

Gibson PH, Coughlin J et al (2002). Self management education and regular practioner review for adults with asthma. Cochrane database of systemic review. Issue 3 CD001117.

Giraud V, Rogeaux Y, Dusser D(2006) Asthma control following initial inhaled corticosteroid monotherapy in mild to moderate asthma : a 4-8 weeks observational study. Respiration.73, 617-622.

Gleeson C. (1998) Asthma Education. How best to deliver it. The Asthma journal Sept.1998, Vol3. Issue 3,126-129.

Global initiative for asthma (GINA, 2006) Global strategy for asthma management and prevention. Revised edition. MRC vision. 30, http:// www.who.int/ respiratory/asthma /GINA_we_2006_copy right%5B1/5D.pdf (last accessed on 13/5/2010

Global initiative for asthma (GINA) 2008. The Gina Report is available on WWW. Ginasthma.org last accessed on 8/6/2010

Higgins PS, Wakefield D, Cloutier MM. Risk Factors for Asthma and Asthma Severity in Nonurban Children in Connecticut. CHEST 2005; 128(6): 3846 -3853.

Holgate ST and Douglass J (2006). Fast Facts: Asthma. Health press.
Oxford ISBN1-903734-54-1.

Holgate S92007) A new approach to asthma management. Practice nursing .18, 6,288-294

.Hoskins G et al (2000). Risk factor and cost associate with asthma attach. Thorax, 55:19-24

Jarvis S (2006) Asthma action plan.practise: what are the needs? Thorax.vol 51, S 13-S 17 nurse.31, 3, 33-38.

John F Price (1996) Issues in Adolescent asthma

Jordan S and white J (2001). Bronchodilators: implications for nursing standards.15, 27, 45-52.

Kelley CF, Mannino DM, Homa DM, Savage-Brown A, Holguin F. Asthma Phenotypes, Risk Factors, and Measures of Severity in a National Sample of US Children. PEDIATRICS. 2005; 115(3):726-731.

Keely D. How to achieve better outcome in treatment of asthma in general practice. BMJ 1993, 307, 1261-1263.

Khadadah, M. Mahboub, B. Al-Busaidi, N.H. Sliman, N. Soriano, J.B. Bahous, J. AIRGEN survey, The International Journal of Tuberculosis and Lung Disease, Volume 13, Number 8, August 2009 , pp. 1015-1022(8)

Kumar P, Clark M (Ed.). Clinical Medicine Fourth Edition. 1998. Harcourt Brace and Company Limited.

Kunzite J, Griška E, Bojarskas J. Time trends in the prevalence of asthma and allergy among 6–7-year-old children. Results from ISAAC phase I and III studies in Kaunas, Lithuania. Medicina (Kaunas) 2008; 44(12): 944-952.

Liebhart J, Malolepszy J, Wojtyniak B, Mickiewicz K, Plusa K, Gladysz U. Prevalence and Risk Factors for Asthma in Poland: Results From the PMSEAD Study .J Investing Allergol Clin Immunol 2007; 17 (6): 367-374.

Levy ML, fletcher M, price DB et al (2006), international primary care respiratory group (IPCRG) Guidelines: diagnosis of respiratory diseases in primary care, primary care respiratory journal.15, 1, 20-34.

Llli S, Von Mutius E, Lau S et al(2001) .early childhood infectious diseases and the development of asthma up to school age. British medical journal.322 (7283), 390-395.

Llli S, Von Mutius E, Lau S et al (2006) Perennial allergen sensitization early in life in children. The lancet.368, 9537, 763-770

Lyte G, Milnes L, Keating P and Finke A(2007) Review management of children with asthma in primary care: a qualitative case study, journal of clinical nursing 16,(7b),123-

Martini F, ober W, Garisson C, Welch K, Hutching R (2006). Fundamentals of anatomy and physiology (7th edition) Chapter 23(The respiratory system). Benjamin Cummings.

Ministry of health UAE. Asthma in United Arab Emirates. [cited on 2/9/2008), available from: URL: http://www.moh.gov.ae/en/Page_573.aspx

Murray JF and Nadel JA.(1994) Textbook of respiratory medicine, W B Saunders, Philadelphia.

Myers T. Guidelines for Asthma Management: A Review and Comparison of 5 Current Guidelines. RESPIRATORY CARE .2008: 53(6): 751- 769.

Newell K (2006) concordance with asthma medication: the nurse's role. Nursing standard.20, 26, 31-33.

Nunn JF (1993). Nuns applied Respiratory physiology. Butterworth Heinemann. Oxford.

Platt-Mills, TEA (2005). Asthma severity and prevalence, an ongoing interaction between exposure, life style and Hygiene. Plos Med 2(2) e34.

Roberts J (2002) the management of poorly controlled asthma. Nursing standard.16, 21, 45-51.

Scullion JE (2005) a proactive approach to asthma. Nursing standard.16, 21, 45-51

Scullion JE (2005b) asthma reviews-what should we measure? Practice Nurse .29, 10, 39-44.

Steven K, Neville RG, Hoskins G (2002) the RPC s Three key questions for asthma: review of practical Use. British journal of community nursing.7, 6,300-303.

Thomas M, Chrystyn J et al (2007) Consensus guideline on the use of inhaler devices in asthma. Medium group publishing limited.

World health organization.2002 Prevention of allergy and allergic asthma. The WHO/WAO Meeting on the prevention of allergy and allergic asthma. Geneva, 8-9 January 2002.

Zandwicz MM (2007) Pharmacology of asthma. American journal of pharmaceutical education.71 (5), 98, 1-12.

edinbburgh.http://www.sign.ac.uk/guidelines/fultex/63/index.html. (Last accessed (11/5/2010).

National asthma council Australia (2006) Asthma management handbooks, drugs and devices (electronic) Last accessed10/1/2011 available at (www. Nationalasthma.org.au.

Bronchial Asthma Care and Control Profile at Primary Healthcare Facilities of Dubai

Ashtar MS.[1], Monsef NA.[1], Buharoun AI.[2], Mubarak Obaid HA.[1], Al Faisal W.[1]*, Hussein H.[1]

[1] Health Affairs Department, Primary Health Care Services Sector, Dubai Health Authority, Dubai, UAE
[2] Health Centres Department, Primary Health Care Services Sector, Dubai Health Authority, Dubai, UAE

* **Corresponding authors:** E-mail address: **wldalfaisal@gmail.com**
msashtar@dha.gov.ae

Key Words: Bronchial asthma, Primary health care, Dubai
Conflict of interest: The authors declare that they do not have any conflict of interest.

Abstract

Background: The morbidity and mortality from asthma appear to be increasing despite changes in medical practice and many advances in treatment of asthma over the years. Most of the deaths are due to relatively acute attacks, although usually against a background of poorly controlled asthma. Many deaths and unnecessary morbidity have been associated with overreliance on bronchodilators, underuse of inhaled and oral corticosteroids, failure to make objective measurements of severity and inadequate supervision.

Objectives: This study is designed to investigate the level of asthma control, percentage of using inhaled corticosteroids, percentage of sick off days because of asthma, percentage of Asthma flow charts implementation (Initial Assessment form & Follow up form), percentage of additional forms implementation (Asthma Action plan Form, Asthma Control Test Form & Self-Management Goals & Plan Form), and percentage of Smokers among asthmatics.

Methods: A retrospective records review of registered asthmatic patients was implemented. All registered asthma patients at primary health care facilities of Dubai Health Authority for the period of 2006-2015 were included in the current audit retrieved from SAM IT registry system. A convenience sample was chosen. It was composed of 476 in 2010, 341 in 2011, 318 in 2012, 188 in 2013, 450 in 2014, and 440 in 2015.

Results: The level of control in 2015 was 53.4% in General Outpatient Department of PHC (OPD) and 64.9% in Bronchial Asthma mini clinics in PHC. The best level was shown in 2014. As for using inhaled corticosteroids, it was shown that it was 82% in OPD clinics while it was 95% in asthma mini clinic cases. The study reflected significant increasing in use of inhaled corticosteroid. No sick off days became about 32% at general OPD clinics, and 42% at asthma mini clinics. Concerning initial Assessment & Follow-up Forms Implementation, the study revealed that they are implemented in 91% of asthma patients treated in general OPD clinics, and in 100% of asthma patients treated in mini clinics. As for additional forms implementation, the study showed that they are implemented in 97% of asthma patients in the mini clinics and 46% of asthma patients in the general outpatient clinics. The study revealed that smoking was reduced to 6.36%.

Conclusion: Improvement of bronchial asthma care was noticed at primary health care settings in Dubai Health Authority. It was clear that managing asthma in mini-clinics setting produced more positive outcomes in terms of control compared to asthma management in general outpatient clinics, based on different outcomes indicators. There are still many gaps that needs to be bridged in asthma management system at primary health care to raise the level of control to a higher standard level, like sticking to asthma management guidelines, health care givers capacity building and developing asthma management care independently. It is recommenced to investigate causes of poor adherence to asthma management in 2015 by primary health care physicians. Addressing gaps will strengthen asthma management care. Adhering to international standards, Continuous professional development and capacity building are factors that are in need to be taken into consideration.

Introduction

It has been evidenced based that bronchial asthma is one of the commonest chronic diseases worldwide. It is also one of the common cause of admission to hospital. There is now ample evidence that prevalence, morbidity and mortality are on the rise.[1-3] Bronchial asthma is considered a "bread and butter issue of clinical practice". Worldwide an estimated 300 million individuals are affected.[4,5]

The morbidity and mortality from asthma appears to be increasing despite changes in medical practice and many advances in treatment of asthma over the years. Most of the deaths are due to relatively acute attacks, although usually against a background of poorly controlled asthma. Many deaths and much unnecessary morbidity have been associated with overreliance on bronchodilators, underuse of inhaled and oral corticosteroids, failure to make objective measurements of severity and inadequate supervision.[6] Several studies have tried to determine why patients die from asthma. Some have looked at the assessment and management of exacerbations of asthma in general practice and hospital.[6] while others have looked at individual deaths from asthma in an attempt to identify factors related to mortality.[6-10] All have suggested that there are deficiencies in both assessment and treatment.

We carried out this medical audit to assess critically the quality of medical care given to patients with asthma in primary health care settings belonging to Dubai health authority. Our aim was to determine whether our patients evaluation and management measured up to the standard recommended guidelines.[11] In this way, if we do find deficiencies in the management compared to the accepted standard then we could implement changes and suggest recommendations. This would serve to improve the delivery of care to asthma patients.

Objectives

This study is designed to investigate the level of asthma control, percentage of using inhaled corticosteroids, percentage of sick off days because of asthma, percentage of Asthma flow charts implementation (Initial Assessment form & Follow up form), percentage of additional forms implementation (Asthma Action plan Form, Asthma Control Test Form & Self-Management Goals & Plan Form), and percentage of Smokers among asthmatics.

Methodology

An Audit study has been carried out at primary health care centers at Dubai Health authority for the period 2006-2015. This audit is conducted in the General Outpatient Department (OPD) and Bronchial Asthma mini clinics. A retrospective records review of registered asthmatic patients was conducted. All registered asthma patients at PHC/DHA for the period of 2006-2015 were included in the current audit retrieved from SAM IT registry system applied at DHA facilities. A convenience sample was chosen. It was composed of 476 in 2010, 341 in 2011, 318 in 2012, 188 in 2013, 450 in 2014, and 440 in 2015. Those who were excluded are: bronchial asthma patients who visit health centers for issues not related to asthma, those with no asthma evaluation at those particular visits, children below 2 years, and patients with Bronchial Asthma receiving asthma care from other health care providers.

Audit Criteria utilized: PHC Bronchial asthma guidelines is used for the comparisons.

- Asthma patients attending PHC should have their asthma controlled as per guideline
- Asthma patients attending PHC should use inhaled corticosteroids as per guidelines
- Asthma patients attending PHC should not have sick off days because of asthma
- Asthma flow charts should be implemented in the files of asthma patients in PHC with proper documentation of:
    - Demographic Data: Age, Sex, Nationality, Marital Status, Occupation & Education
    - Clinical Data: Smoking Status, Family History of Bronchial Asthma, Classification, Triggers, Pick Flow Rate (PEFR), Night Symptoms, Use of Inhaled Corticosteroids, sick off day
- Asthma Additional Forms (Asthma action plan/Asthma control Test/ Self-management goals & plan forms) should be implemented in the files of asthma patients in PHC
- Asthma patients attending PHC should be non-smokers

Audit Standards

- > 45% of Asthma patients attending PHC should have their asthma controlled as per guidelines by 31st Dec 2015
- > 70% of Asthma patients attending PHC should use ICS by 31st Dec 2015
- > 50% of Asthma patients attending PHC should not have sick off days because of asthma by 31st Dec 2015

- >95% of the files of asthma patients in PHC should have Asthma flow charts implemented with proper documentation by 31st Dec 2015
- >65% of the files of asthma patients in PHC should have Asthma Additional Forms implemented by 31st Dec 2015 (First year audited 2015)
- >95% of Asthma patients attending PHC should be non-smokers by 31st Dec 2015

Auditing Tool

Structured auditing tool was used and included domains of socio-demographic data, quality of care & asthma control measurements, and implementation of forms.

Results

Figures 1, 2 and 3 show the level of control. The level of control in 2015 was 53.4% in OPD and 64.9% in mini clinic. The best level was shown in 2014.

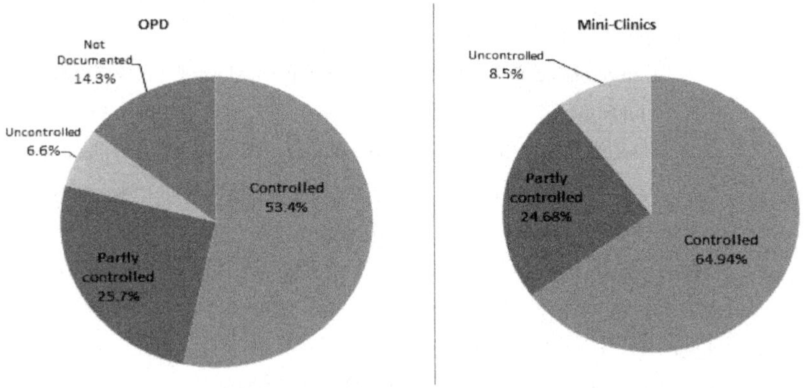

Figure 1: Classification of registerd asthma cases at PHC according to the level of control on 2015

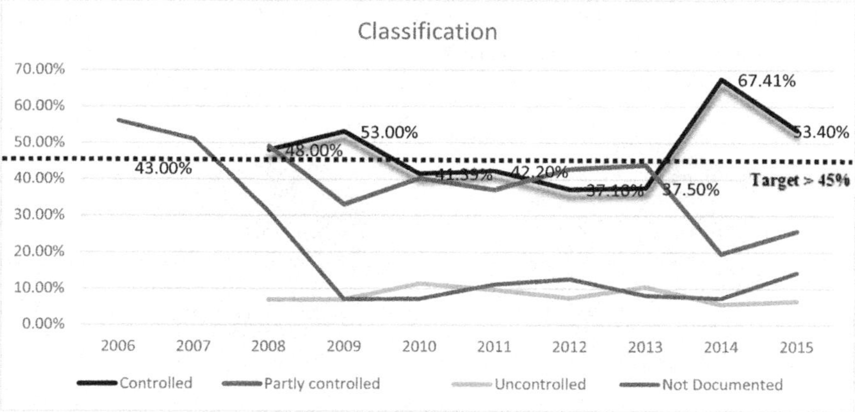

Figure 2: Frequency distribution of PHC registered asthma cases based on Level of Control Classification (2006-2015)

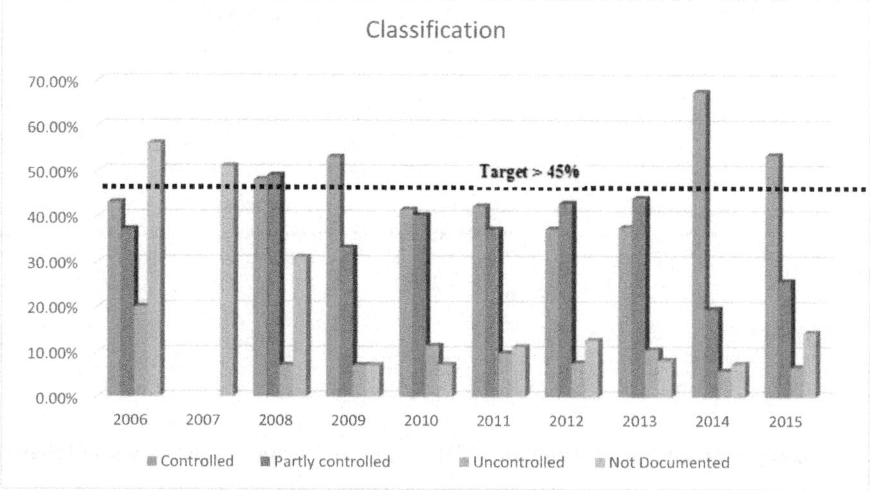

Figure 3: Frequency distribution of PHC registered asthma cases based on Level of Control Classification (2006-2015)

The rate of prescribing Inhaled Corticosteroids was 95% among asthma mini clinic cases, and 82% among general outpatient clinics. The study reflected significant increasing in use of inhaled corticosteroid, figures (4 and 5).

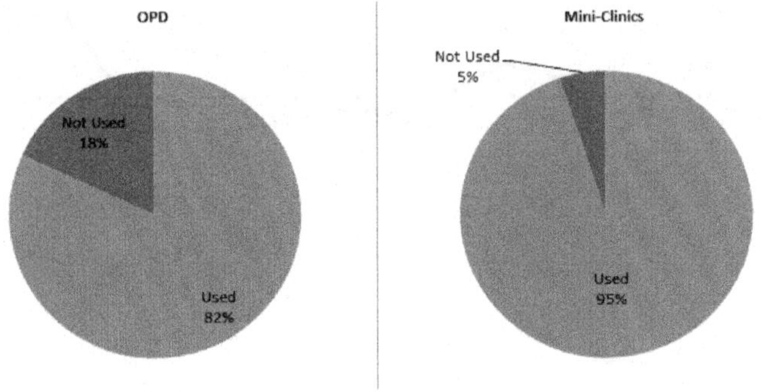

Figure 4: Frequency distribution of asthma cases based on Use of Inhaled Corticosteroids (2015)

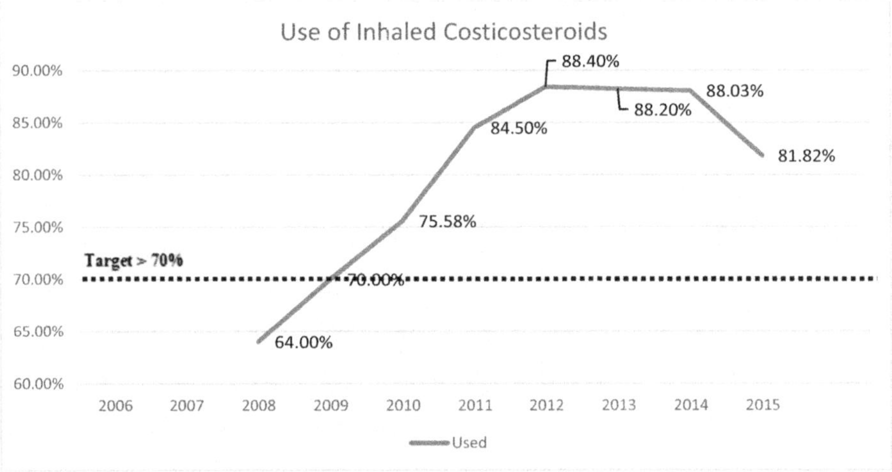

Figure 5: Frequency distribution of PHC registered asthma based on Use of Inhaled Corticosteroids (2006-2015)

Figures 6, 7 and 8 show data about reducing sick off days because of asthma. The study showed that by the end of 2015 the percentage of asthma patients with no asthma sick off days was about 32% in general outpatient clinic Vis 42% in mini clinics. Best results was 85% in 2011.

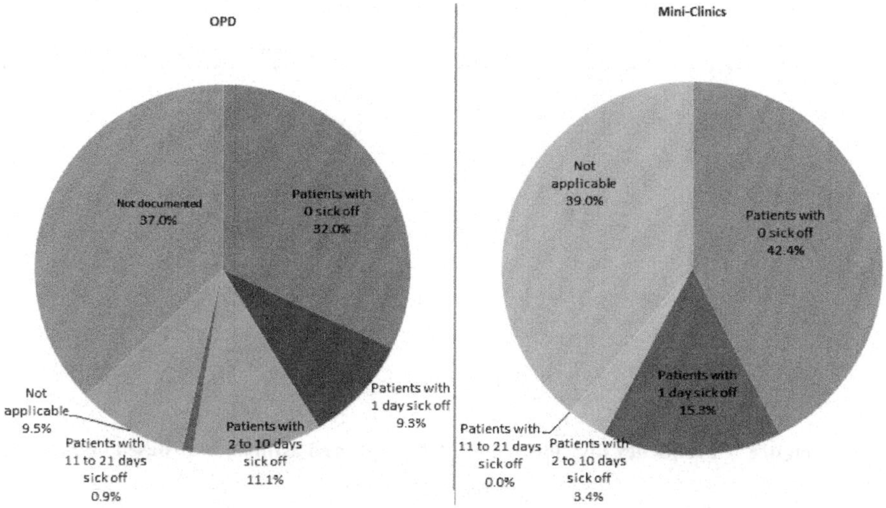

Figure 6: Frequency distribution of PHC registered asthma cases based on Sick off Days 2015

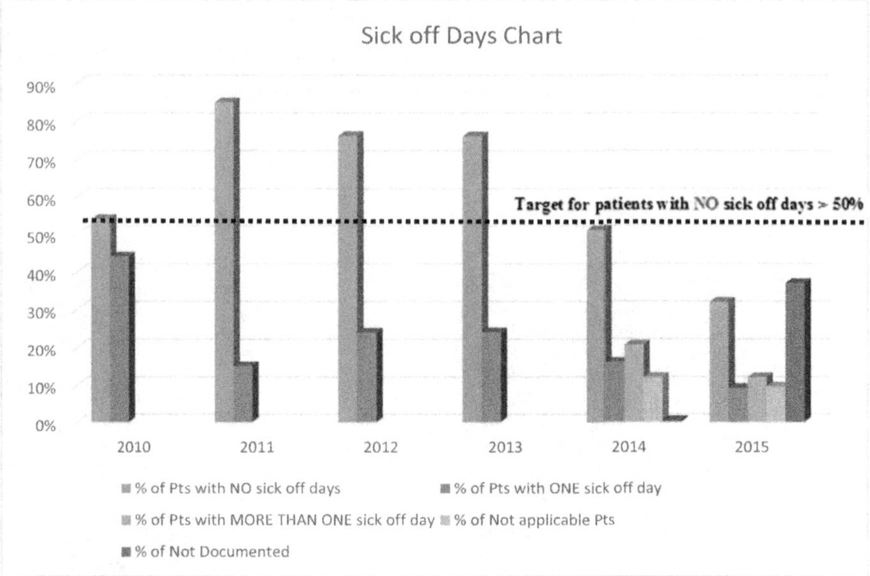

Figure 7: Frequency distribution of PHC registered asthma cases based on Sick off Days (2010-2015)

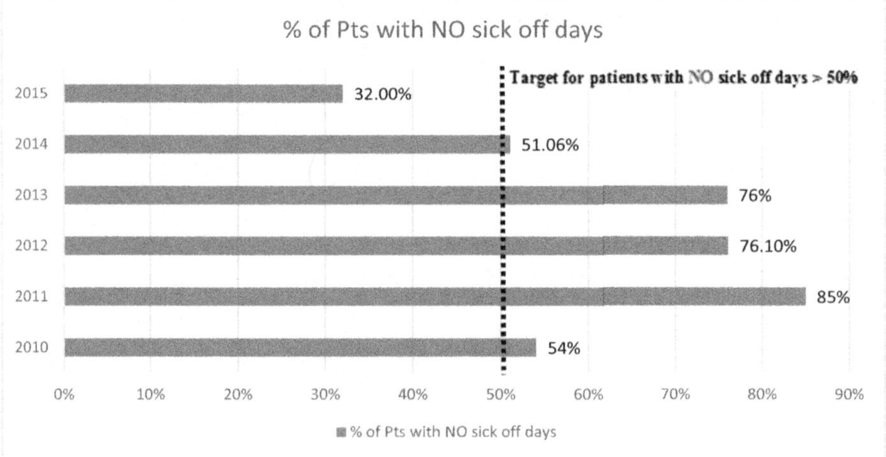

Figure 8: Frequency distribution of PHC registered asthma cases based on percentage of patients with no sick off days (2010-2015)

Concerning initial assessment and follow-up forms implementation, the current study revealed that implementation is 100% in asthma mini clinic and about 91% in general outpatient clinics by the end of 2015. Regarding additional forms implementation which started in 2014, the study showed that they were implemented in 46% of patients in general outpatient's clinics and in 97% in asthma mini clinics by the end of 2015 (figures 9, 10 and 11).

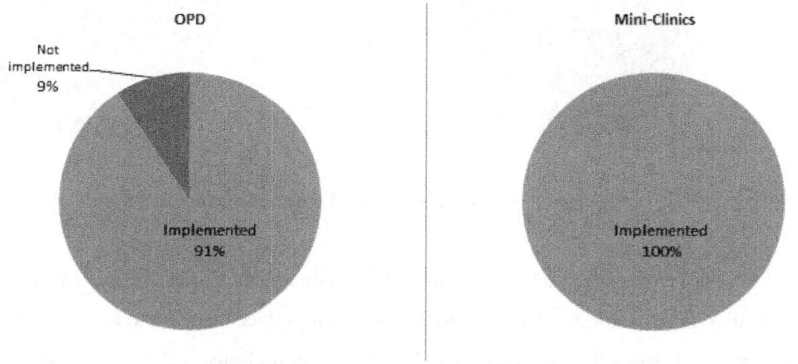

Figure 9: Frequency distribution of PHC registered Asthma cases based on Initial Assessment & Follow-up Forms Implementation 2015

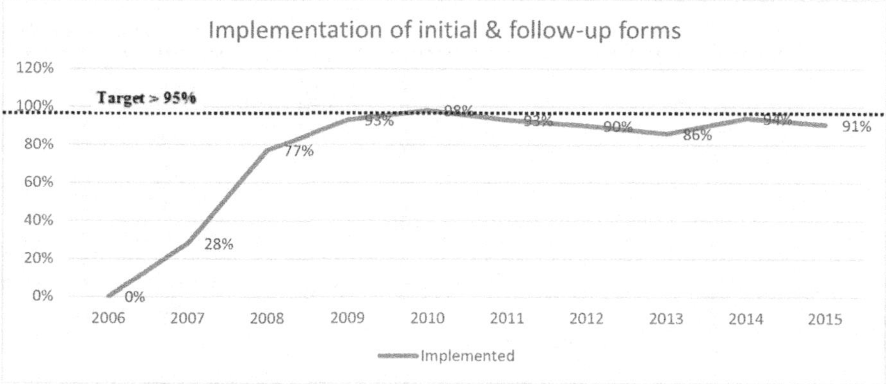

Figure 10: Initial Assessment and Follow-up Forms Implementation (2006-2015)

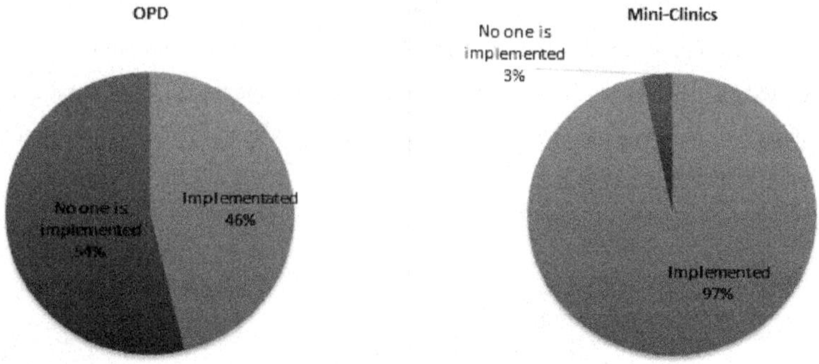

Figure 11: Additional Forms Implementation 2015

The study revealed that smoking was totally reduced to 6.36% by the end of 2015. Although target is not generally reached, which is to reduce smokers to less than 5%, The percentage of smokers was reduced to 2% in the mini-clinics and to 6% in the general outpatient clinics figures (12 and 13).

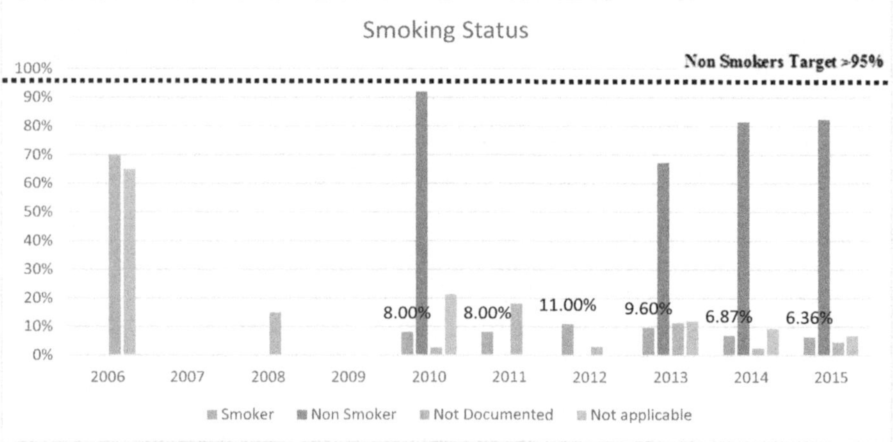

Figure 12: Frequency distribution of PHC registered asthma cases based on Smoking Status for the period (2010-2015)

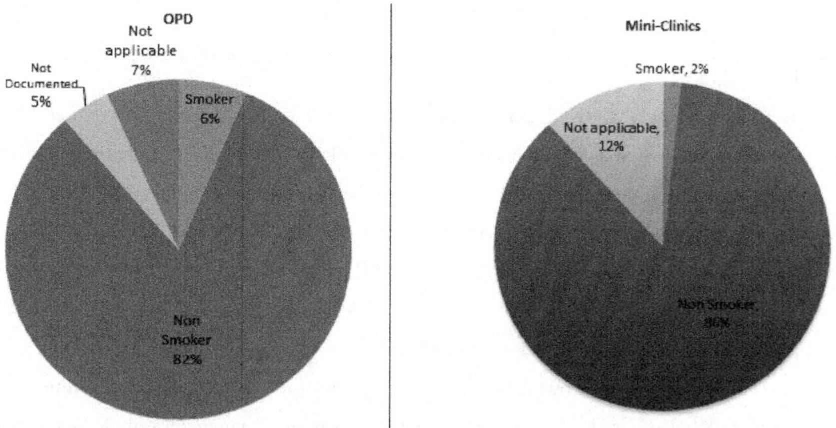

Figure 13: Frequency distribution of asthma cases based on Smoking Status (2015)

The study showed that asthma management in asthma mini-clinics was significantly effective compared to asthma management in general outpatient clinic:

- In level of control (64.94% Vis 53.4%)
- In prescribing ICS (82% Vis 95%)
- In reducing sick off days (32% Vis 42% with no sick off days)
- In initial assessment and follow up forms implementation (100% Vis 91%)
- In additional forms implementation (46% Vis 97%).
- In reducing smoking (2% Vis 6% non-smokers)

As per comparing 2014 and 2015 asthma control results, the study revealed the following results:

- Decrease in level of control from 67.41 to 53.40
- Decrease in use of ICS form 88% to 81%
- Decease of zero sick off days from 51% to 32%

- Decrease of initial assessment and follow up forms implementation from 94% to 91%
- Decrease of additional forms implementation from 65% to 45%

Discussion

The current study showed that in 2014 almost 67% of total asthmatic patients were classified controlled as per levels of asthma control criteria in GINA guidelines 2015.[5] this is significantly higher than results of other studies. One study conducted in USA in 2007 showed that only 50% of adults and 62.6% of children have controlled asthma all over USA. Another one conducted in Malaysia in 2011 showed that only 39.2 % of the patients were classified as having controlled asthma, 34.3 % had asthma that was partly controlled and 26.5 % of the patients had uncontrolled asthma.[12-14]

Current study showed that patients attending asthma management clinic (mini-clinics) revealed better control results regarding asthma management outcomes compared to patients attending general outpatient clinics. These results were similar to other studies that concluded the level of control of bronchial asthma was significantly better among patients attending asthma clinics than those attending general clinics, and females were found to have significantly better control compared to males.[15-18]

Current study showed that medical records or asthma management and follow up documentation was significantly improved along years of implementing standardized asthma management care at Primary health care services. Percentage of documentation in OPD clinics versus mini-clinics in 2015 was as the following: 90% and 100% for occupation; 91% in both for education level; 95% and 100% for smoking status; 90% and 100% for family history of bronchial asthma; 87% and 100% for trigger factors; 88% and 100% for night symptom; 88% and 98% for peak flow readings; 86% and 100% for diagnostic classification; 100% in both for medicine prescription; and 63% and 100% for sick off days. This was contradicted with similar studies[19-22] which stated low documentation levels, for example, documentation of clinical assessment in other studies was low for previous admissions (2%), rescue nebulization (25%), duration of symptoms (57%), trigger factors (19%), compliance (9%), clinical signs (48%), peak flow rate (3%), and inhaler technique (5%). The diagnosis of asthma exacerbation was documented in 77%

of the episodes. Documentation of therapy was also low (3% for oxygen therapy and 24% for systemic steroids). Documentation of post-nebulization assessment, follow-up appointment, and referral to asthma clinic were found in 37%, 23% and 11% of cases respectively. No documented evidence was found for referral to chest specialist or spirometry.

The current study managed to identify a gap of poor adherence to asthma management guidelines by primary health care physicians in 2014 which led to a decrease in asthma control level in 2015 compared to 2014. Other similar studies showed that 8% of primary health care physicians had good theoretical knowledge of bronchial asthma, and 41% had poor knowledge. The knowledge of the residents was better than that of the PHC physicians in the same study. The mean knowledge score was significantly better among those using guidelines compared to the rest. About 23% had good knowledge of inhaler techniques. Knowledge of PHC physicians and FM residents about dry powder inhalers was deficient, and PHC physicians had little knowledge of metered dose inhalers with spacers.[23, 24]

Conclusion

Improvement of bronchial asthma care was noticed at primary health care settings in Dubai Health Authority. It was clear that managing asthma in mini-clinics setting produced more positive outcomes in terms of control compared to asthma management in general outpatient clinics, based on different outcomes indicators. There are still many gaps that needs to be bridged in asthma management system at primary health care to raise the level of control to a higher standard level, like sticking to asthma management guidelines, health care givers capacity building and developing asthma management care independently. It is recommenced to investigate causes of poor adherence to asthma management in 2015 by primary health care physicians. Addressing gaps will strengthen asthma management care. Adhering to international standards, Continuous professional development and capacity building are factors that are in need to be taken into consideration.

References

1. Bumey, P. Asthma mortality in England and Wales. Evidence for a further. Increase 1974-84. Lancet, 1986;ii:323-6.
2. Flemming. D.M. and Crombie, D.L. Prevalence of asthma and hay fever in England and Wales. Br. Med. J., 1987; 294:279-83.
3. M'Hchell, E.A. Increasing prevalence of asthma in children, N.Z. Med. J., 1983;96:463-4
4. Partrige MR, van der Molen T, Myrseth SE et al. Attitudes and actions of asthma patients on regular maintenance therapy: the INSPIRE STUDY. *BMC Pulmonary Medicine* 2006; **6**: 13.
5. Usha Devi B, Hairul Izwan AR, Munjeet KPS, Rosidah CP. An Audit of Bronchial Asthma Control at a Primary Public Health Care Facility. Malaysian Journal of Public Health Medicine 2011, Vol. 11(2): 22-26
6. British Thoracic Society. Guidelines on bronchial asthma. Br Med J 1993; 306: 776-982.
7. Bucknall CE, Robertson C, Moron F, Stevenson RD. Management of asthma in hospital: a prospective audit. Br Med J 1988; 296: 1637-9.
8. Bucknall CE, Robertson C, Moron F, Stevenson RD. References in hospital asthma management. Lancet i 1988; 748-50.
9. Dason, Maclove HL. Controlled investigation of deaths from asthma in hospital in the North East Thomas region. Br Med J 1987; 294: 1255-8.
10. British Thoracic Association: Death from asthma in two regions of England Br Med J 1982; 285: 1251-5.
11. British Thoracic Society, Guidelines Qn the management of asthma. Thorax, 1993; 48(250 ppl): S 1-524.
12. Juniper EF, Bousquet J, Abetz L et al. Identifying "well-controlled" and "not well-controlled" asthma using Asthma Controlled Questionnaire. Respiratory Medicine 2006; 100: 616-624
13. Guidelines on management of adult asthma: a consensus statement of the Malaysian Thoracic Society. Medical Journal of Malaysia 1996; 51(1): 114-128.

14. CDC. Asthma Stats. National Asthma Education and Prevention Program Expert panel - report 3 2007. Available from: http://www.cdc.gov/asthma/asthma_stats/uncontrolled_asthma.pdf. Accessed 3 March 2016
15. Wesaam Ghafouri, Homied Al-Omari, Mohammed Bakhatma. Control levels among asthmatic patients attending asthma clinic at Eskan PHC center and general clinic at Kakiah PHC center, Makkah Al - Mukarramah, Saudi Arabia. Int J Med Sci Public Health. 2014; 3(1): 89-95doi: 10.5455/ijmsph.2013.151020131,
16. Wechsler ME. Managing asthma in primary care: Putting new guideline recommendations into context. Mayo Clin Proc. 2009; 84:707-17.
17. Bateman ED, Hurd SS, Barnes PJ, Bousquet J, Drazen JM, FitzGerald M, et al. Global strategy for asthma management and prevention: GINA executive summary. Eur Respir J. 2008; 31(1):143-78.
18. Abudahish A, Bella H. Primary care physician's perceptions and practices on asthma care in Aseer region, Saudi Arabia. Saudi Med J. 2006; 27:333-7.
19. Sawsan A Baddar, Aida I Al-Ismaili, Muna A Al-Taie, Abdulaziz M Al-Mahrezi, and Omar A Al-Rawas. Documentation of the Management of Asthma Exacerbation in Adults by Primary Health Care Physicians in a Teaching Hospital in Oman. Sultan Qaboos Univ Med J. 2010 Dec; 10(3): 335–340. Published online 2010 Nov 14. PMCID: PMC3074746
20. Barnes PJ. Asthma guidelines: recommendations versus reality. Respir Med. 2004; 98:S1-7.
21. Miller MK, Lee JH, Miller DP, Wenzel SE. TENOR Study Group. Recent asthma exacerbations: a key predictor of future exacerbations. Respir Med. 2007; 101:481–9.
22. Wisnivesky JP, Lorenzo J, Lyn-Cook R, Newman T, Aponte A, Kiefer E, et al. Barriers to adherence to asthma management guidelines among inner-city primary care providers. Ann Allergy Asthma Immunol. 2008; 101:264–70.
23. Haneen A. Yousef, Manal Koura, and Abdullah A. Yousef. Knowledge about bronchial asthma management in primary health care physicians in Al-Khobar City,

Saudi Arabia. Family Community Med. 2015 Jan-Apr; 22(1): 1–7. doi: 10.4103/2230-8229.149567PMCID: PMC4317988

24. Grant EN, Moy JN, Turner-Roan K, Daugherty SR, Weiss KB. Asthma care practices, perceptions, and beliefs of Chicago-area primary-care physicians. Chicago Asthma Surveillance Initiative Project Team. Chest. 1999; 116:145S–54.

Epidemiological profile and Clinical Characteristics of the Childhood Asthma among School Students in Dubai, UAE

AlBehandy NS,[1] Hussein H,[1] Al Faisal W,[1] El Sawaf E,[2] Wasfy A,[2] Alshareef N,[1] Altheeb AAS,[1]

[1] School and Educational Institutions Health Unit, Health Affars Department, Primary Health Care Services Sector, Dubai Health Authority.

[2] Staff Development, Health Centers Department. Primary Health Care Services Sector, Dubai Health Authority

Key Words: Childhood Asthma, profile, Dubai

Conflict of interest: The authors declare that they don't have any conflict of interest.

Correspondence to: Dr. Hamid Hussain: hyhussain@dha.gov.ae

Abstract:

Background: Prevalence Asthma has wide variations. It is the most common chronic disease facing the childhood in the first world countries. Globally, epidemiologic data estimate that nearly 300 million people worldwide suffer from asthma with expectation that this number will grow by more than 100 million by 2025. Annually 250,000 deaths are attributed to this disease. With approximately 500,000 hospitalizations per year and 13 million missed school days. Asthma is the third-ranking cause of hospitalization among children under 15 In the UAE.**Objectives:** To study the prevalence, clinical and epidemiological profile, and socio demographic risk factors of the childhood asthma in Dubai. **Methodology:** A cross-sectional study was conducted among students in preparatory and secondary schools "Governmental and Private" in Dubai, U.A.E. A sample of 1639 students was selected randomly by multistage stratified random sampling technique. **Results:** 16.7% have had an asthma attack at some point of time. About 38.5% had asthma at age of less than 3 years, 28.6% from 3 to less than 6 years, 19% from 6 to less than 9 years and only 13.9% at an age of 9 years or more with a mean of 5.0 ± 2.9 years. Most of the studied students had no wheezing or whistling in the chest at any time in the past (83.5 while 72.9% had wheezes within the last 12 months. Amongst those who had wheezes in the last 12 months 59.8% had 1 to less than 4 attacks during this period, 23.6% had 4 to 12 attacks and 8.5% had more than 12 attacks. As regards the frequency of asthma symptoms per week it can be noted that 8.5% had the symptoms over the day, another 11.1% had daily symptoms, 49.2% had the symptoms 2 times or less / week and another 31.2% had the symptoms frequency of more than 2 times / week but not daily. Regarding the sleeping it was disturbed less than once weekly in 35.2% while it was disturbed once or more per week in 19.1%. Studying the frequency of nocturnal symptoms; 6.5% had frequent nocturnal symptoms, 11.1% had these symptoms more than once per week, 20.1% experienced the nocturnal symptoms 3-4 times a month and the vast majority experienced the symptoms less than twice monthly. Speech limitation due to wheezing was reported by 42.2%, and 66.8% experienced wheezes during and after exercise. As regards using inhalers, the frequency of use ranged from less than or twice weekly in 57.8% and several times/ day in 8%, while it was used daily in 8.5% and used more than twice weekly in 25.6%. **Conclusion:** The prevalence of asthma among secondary school student in Dubai is high. Early onset of asthmatic attacks was clearly eminent among the study sample where 67.1% of them had their first attacks before six years old with a mean age of 5.0 ± 2.9 years for onset of the first attacks. Although Boys had higher statistically significant propensity to acquire bronchial asthma, gender revealed no difference concerning severity. Emirian students and those in governmental schools were more affected with bronchial asthma. Although apparently higher among low educated mothers, illiterate fathers had statistically significant higher percentage of asthmatic children. **Recommendations:** A national asthma surveillance system should be developed in order to early detect and manage bronchial asthma among schoolchildren.

Introduction

Bronchial asthma is defined as a chronic, inflammatory lung disease, which characteristically presents by cough, dyspnea, wheezing and chest tightness, which occurs in paroxysms and is usually related to specific triggering events involving partial or complete reversible airway narrowing plus increased airways responsiveness to a variety of stimuli. [1] Asthma and obesity are recently evolved into two major public health concerns in developed countries.[2] Asthma prevalence exists globally in wide variations.[3] It is the most common chronic disease facing the childhood in first world countries. Recurrent asthma-like symptoms were reported in approximately 32 percent of preschool children in the United States and Europe.[4] Globally, epidemiologic data estimate that nearly 300 million people worldwide suffer from asthma with expectation that this number will grow by more than 100 million by 2025. Annually 250,000 deaths are attributed to this disease.[5] with approximately 500,000 hospitalizations per year and 13 million missed school days.[6] Asthma is the third-ranking cause of hospitalization among children under 15.[7] In the UAE, in Alain area a study held between 2007- 2010 showed that the prevalence of asthma in the study group aged 13-19 years was 16%, while that in the adult group 19 years and above was 12%.[8]

Asthma is a large and growing threat to children's health and well-being.[1] It affects 5-10% of the population or an estimated 23.4 million persons, including 7 million children in the U.S.[9] Asthma is the most common chronic disease of childhood. Almost 1 in 8 school-aged children are affected by asthma, and 10% of children (compared with 5% of adults) take medication for it.[10,11] Worldwide, an estimated 300 million people are affected by asthma. Based on the application of standardized methods to the measurement of the prevalence of asthma and wheezing illness in children and adults, it appears that the global prevalence of asthma ranges 1-18% of the population in different countries.[5] There is a good evidence that international differences in asthma symptom prevalence have been reduced, particularly in the age 13-14 year age group, with decrease in prevalence in North America and Western Europe and increase prevalence in regions where prevalence was previously low. Although there was little change in the overall prevalence of current wheeze, the percentage of children reported to have had asthma increased significantly, possibly reflecting greater awareness of this condition and/or changes in diagnostic practice. The increases in asthma symptoms prevalence in Africa, Latin America and parts of Asia indicate that the global burden of asthma is continuing to rise, but the global prevalence differences are lessening.[12] Asthma is a leading chronic illness among children and youth in the United States. In 2007, 5.6 million school-aged children and youth (5-17 years old) were reported to currently have asthma; and 2.9 million had an asthma episode or attack within the previous year. On average, in a classroom of 30 children, about 3 are likely to have asthma.[13] In a study done in Egypt in 2009 the overall prevalence of asthma among school children was 7.7% (8% in urban areas and 7% in rural areas).[14] In a study conducted in State of Qatar, the school children aged from 6-14 year revealed a prevalence of bronchial asthma as high as 19.8 % in 2004.[15] In between 2007-2009 in Saudi Arabia (Riyadh), a study among the same age range (6-14) revealed that the prevalence of asthma among school children was 11.4% [16] while in Oman, the prevalence of asthma reached 10.5% and 20.7% in 6-7 and 13-14 years old Omani children respectively.[17]

The World Health Organization (WHO) has estimated that 15 million disability-adjusted life-years are lost annually due to asthma, representing 1% of the total global disease burden Annual worldwide deaths from asthma have been estimated at 250,000 and mortality does not appear to correlate well with prevalence. There are insufficient data to fully explain the variations in prevalence within and between populations. Although from the perspective of both the patient and society the cost to control asthma seems high, the cost of not treating asthma correctly is even higher. [5]

Children with asthma are at an increased risk of experiencing asthma-related respiratory symptoms in adult life. [18] Asthma is one of the leading causes of school absenteeism. In 2003, an estimated 12.8 million school days were missed due to asthma among more than 4 million children who reported at least one asthma attack in the preceding year.[19] Low-income populations, minorities, and children living in inner cities experience more emergency department visits, hospitalizations, and deaths due to asthma than the general population.[20] Two old studies on 1994 and 2000 in the UAE among students aged 6-13 showed that the prevalence of asthma was 13,6 % [21] and 13 % [22] respectively. In a recent study in the UAE, in Alain area which was held between 2007-2010 showed that the prevalence of asthma in the group aged 13-19 years was 16%, while that in the adult group 19 years and above was 12 %.[8]

Since Bronchial asthma constitutes an important health problem worldwide related with significant impact in terms of morbidity and mortality, being with allergic rhinitis, the most frequent childhood chronic diseases, showing also a prevalence increase in developed and developing countries, and similarly expected at UAE, this study designed to mapping childhood asthma in Dubai.

Objectives

To study the prevalence, clinical and epidemiological profile, and socio-demographic risk factors of childhood asthma in Dubai.

Methodology

This is a cross sectional study, conducted among students in preparatory and secondary schools "Governmental and Private" in Dubai, U.A.E. Computer program EPI-Info version "6.04" was used for calculation of the minimum sample size required. According to a recent study[8] the prevalence of asthma among adolescent in the UAE was found to be 16%, using 3% degree of precision, 95% confidence interval and 1.5% design effect, the minimum sample size required was 855. A list of schools was obtained from the knowledge and Human Development Authority. Dubai includes 183 school spread along two large districts, Bur Dubai and Diera. Bur Dubai includes 90 schools, 69 private and 21 governmental, where Diera includes 93 schools, 72 private and 21 governmental. The numbers of students in preparatory and secondary stages are 42819 and 34299 respectively. Around 20289 of them in governmental schools, while 56829 are in private schools. This gives a total of 77118 students in both regions (private and governmental). A multistage stratified random sample was used. The strata were based upon geographical districts(Bur-Dubai and Diera), type of schools (governmental or private),educational grade (7th through 12th) and sex (males and females). The number of the governmental schools was less than that of private schools (42 and 141 respectively). According to the numbers of schools, a proportional allocation technique was used to determine the required sample size. 16 private schools (8 from Bur Dubai and 8 from Diera), with 4 schools of boys and 4 schools of girls for each district were randomly selected. Also, 4 governmental schools (2 from Bur Dubai and 2 from Diera), with one school for each gender from each district were randomly selected. From each school one class was selected randomly from each educational grade. All the students in the selected classes were invited to participate in the study and all of them agreed to participate (response rate 100%). The total sample size reached 1639 students.

Results

Table (1) shows the prevalence of asthma among the school students. It showed that 16.7% have had an asthma attack at some point of time.

Table (1): Distribution of preparatory and secondary school students in Dubai according to asthma status, 2011

Asthma status	No.	%
Asthmatic	273	16.7
Non asthmatic	1366	83.3
Total number of students	1639	100

In table (2) asthmatics were classified according to the age of onset of asthma attack, 38.5% had asthma at age of less than 3 years, 28.6% from 3 to less than 6 years, 19% from 6 to less than 9 years and only 13.9% at an age of 9 years or more with a mean of 5.0 ± 2.9 years.

Table (2): Distribution of asthmatic preparatory and secondary school students according to their age at onset of asthma (Dubai, 2011)

Age at onset of asthma (years)	No.	%
<3	105	38.5
3-	78	28.6
6-	52	19.0
9+	38	13.9
Total Number of Students	273	100

In table (3), most of the studied students had no wheezing or whistling in the chest at any time in the past (83.5%), and among the remaining students 72.9% had wheezes within the last 12 months. Amongst those who had wheezes in the last 12 months 59.8% had 1 to less than 4 attacks during this period, 23.6% had 4 to 12 attacks and 8.5% had more than 12 attacks. As regards the frequency of asthma symptoms per week it can be noted that 8.5% had the symptoms over the day, another 11.1% had daily symptoms, 49.2% had the symptoms 2 times or less / week and another 31.2% had the symptoms frequency of more than 2 times / week but not daily. Regarding the sleeping it was disturbed less than once weekly in 35.2% while it was disturbed once or more per week in 19.1%. Studying the frequency of nocturnal symptoms; 6.5% had frequent nocturnal symptoms, 11.1% had these symptoms more than once per week, 20.1% experienced the nocturnal symptoms 3-4 times a month and the vast majority experienced the symptoms less than twice monthly. Speech limitation due to wheezing was reported by 42.2%, and 66.8% experienced wheezes during and after exercise. As regards using inhalers, the frequency of use ranged from less than or twice weekly in 57.8% and several times/ day in 8%, while it was used daily in 8.5% and used more than twice weekly in 25.6%.

Table (3): Distribution of preparatory and secondary school students according to asthma symptoms (Dubai, 2011)

Symptom	No.	%
Wheezing ever*		
No	1366	83.3
Yes	273	16.7
Wheezing within the last 12 months**		
No	74	27.1
Yes	199	72.9
No. of attacks of wheezing within the last 12 months***		
No	16	8.0
1-	119	59.8
4-	47	23.6
>12	17	8.5
Frequency of asthma symptoms/week***		
≤ 2/week	98	49.2
< 2/week but not daily	62	31.2
Daily	22	11.1
Over the day	17	8.5
Sleep disturbance due to wheezing***		
No	91	45.7
less than 1/week	70	35.2
1 or more/week	38	19.1
Frequency of nocturnal symptoms***		

≤ 2/month	124	62.3
3-4 times/month	40	20.1
More than 1/week but not nightly	22	11.1
Frequent (often 7days/week)	13	6.5
Speech limitation due to wheezing***		
No	115	57.8
Yes	84	42.2
Wheezing during or after exercise***		
No	66	33.2
Yes	133	66.8
Rate of inhaler use***		
≤ 2/week	115	57.8
> 2/week but not daily	51	25.6
Daily	17	8.5
Several times/day	16	8.0

**Number of students=1639*

*** Number of asthmatic students=273*

****Number of students with asthma in the last 12 months=199*

Table (4) presents the prevalence of asthma among the studied preparatory and secondary school students according to their demographic characteristics. Considering the age of students, the prevalence of asthma was nearly equal among the different age groups with slight increase in the older age groups. As regards the sex the prevalence of asthma was 1.3 times higher among males compared to females and this was found to be statistically significant. The prevalence according to nationality was 1.4 times higher among locals compared to non-locals and 1.7 times higher among students in governmental than those in private school types and both were statistically significant.

Table (4): Prevalence of asthma among preparatory and secondary school students according to their demographic characteristics (Dubai, 2011)

Characteristic	Total (1639)	Non-asthmatic (1366)		Asthmatic (273)		OR (95%CI)
		No.	%	No.	%	
Age						
11-	433	374	84.4	69	15.6	1
13-	573	477	83.2	96	16.8	1.1 (0.78-1.5)
15-	560	465	83.0	95	17.0	1.1 (0.78-1.6)
17+	63	50	79.4	13	20.6	1.4 (0.73-2.7
Sex						
Female	838	715	85.3	123	14.7	1
Male	801	651	81.3	150	18.8	1.3 (1.0-1.7)
Nationality						
Non Local	776	665	85.7	111	14.3	1
Local	863	701	81.2	162	18.8	1.4 (1.1-1.8)

School type						
Private	1264	1076	85.1	188	14.9	1
Governmental	375	290	77.3	85	22.7	1.7 (1.3-2.3)

Table (5) shows the parental education, crowding index and number of windows per room. It can be noted that as regards father education the highest prevalence of asthma was seen among students whose fathers were of lower education (illiterate 26.7%) as compared to those whose fathers were of university education (15.3%) with the exception of those in preparatory school (14.3%). Students whose fathers were secondary educated had a significant risk of 1.4 times more than those whose fathers were university educated and 2.1 times higher for those whose fathers were illiterate than those whose fathers were university educated. As for the mother education, it can be noted that with the exception of the illiterate group, the prevalence increased with decreased educational level of the mother however the risk was not significant. Crowding index showed no significant association with asthma. As regards the room ventilation (number of windows in the room), the prevalence was found to increase with the decrease of number of windows however this was not significant.

Table (8): Prevalence of asthma among preparatory and secondary school students according to their family and housing characteristics (Dubai, 2011)

Characteristic	Total no. (1639)	Non Asthmatic (n=1366)		Asthmatic (n=273)		OR (95%CI)
		No.	%	No.	%	
Father's Educational level						
University	1062	899	84.7	163	15.3	1
Secondary	321	257	80.1	64	19.9	1.4 (1.0-1.9)*
Preparatory	133	114	85.7	19	14.3	0.9 (0.56-1.5)
Primary	78	63	80.8	15	19.2	1.3 (0.72-2.4)
Illiterate	45	33	73.3	12	26.7	2.1 (1.1-4.0)*
Mother's educational level						
University	855	715	83.6	140	16.4	1
Secondary	424	358	84.4	66	15.6	1.0 (0.67-1.3)
Preparatory	127	102	80.3	25	19.7	1.3 (0.77-2.0)
Primary	137	109	79.6	28	20.4	1.3 (0.83-2.1)
Illiterate	96	82	85.4	14	14.6	0.83 (0.48-1.6)
Crowding index (person\room)						
< 2	1209	998	82.5	211	17.5	1
2-	412	353	85.7	59	14.3	0.74(0.57-1.1)
5+	18	15	83.3	3	16.7	0.94(0.17-3.4)
No. of windows in room						
No	62	55	88.7	7	11.3	1
>2	307	258	84.0	49	16.0	1.5 (0.63-3.4)
≤2	1270	1053	82.9	217	17.1	1.6 (0.72-3.6)

*$P<0.05$

Figure (1) shows the distribution of asthmatic children according to the severity of asthma, it can be noted that 73.3% showed intermittent asthma, 20.1% were classified as mild persistent asthma and only 6.6% were considered moderate and severe persistent asthma. However due to the small sample size among moderate and severe persistent asthma they were combined to the mild persistent asthma group and thus asthmatic students were classified as with either intermittent or persistent asthma for subsequent analysis.

Figure (1): Distribution of asthmatic preparatory and secondary school students according to asthma severity in Dubai, 2011

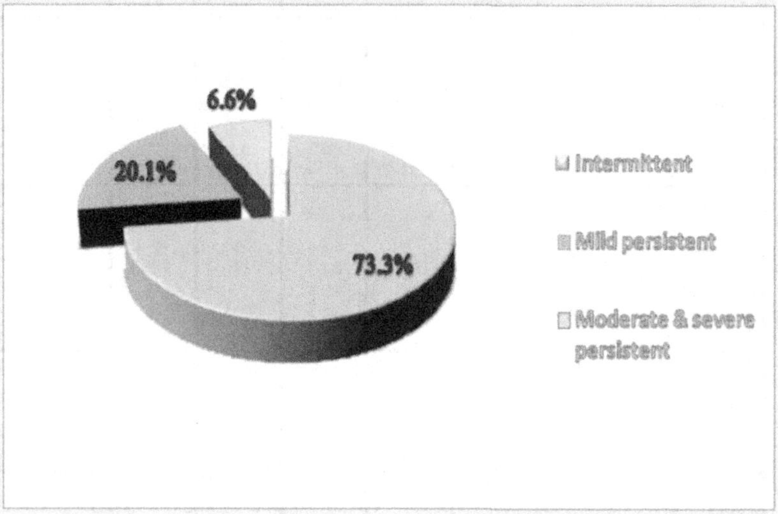

Discussions :

Considering bronchial asthma, it was brought out that 16.7% of the study students have had an asthmatic attack at some point of time with ever complaining of chest wheeze where near three fourths of them complained of this wheeze during the past 12 months prior to the research. This was in compliance with another study done in Alain city in UAE 2009, where the prevalence of asthma was 16 % among group aged 13-19 years old.[8] Another two studies at the years 1994 and 2000 in the UAE among students aged 6-13 years old, showed that the prevalence of asthma was 13,6%[21] and 13 % [22] respectively. When comparing with gulf and some other neighbor countries in the region, asthma prevalence was higher in State of Qatar (19.8%) [15] and Oman (20%), [17] while it was lower in Saudi Arabia (11.4%) [16] and Egypt (7.7 %). [14]

Although the prevalence of asthma was nearly equal among the different age groups, early onset of asthmatic attacks was clearly eminent among the study sample where 67.1% of them had their first attacks before six years old with a mean age of 5.0 $\pm$ 2.9 years for onset of the first attacks. This result comes in consistence with another study done in China which showed that median age of onset of asthma symptoms was 3 years old with peak between 1 to 3 years and more than 90% of children had their onset of asthma before the age of 6 as in our study. [23] Our study showed that the prevalence of persistent asthma among asthmatic students was higher among the older age groups with a very high significant elevated risk among students aged 17 years and older. This is in contrast with another case control study, which was conducted in Baghdad among primary school children aged 6-12 years both showed a decreasing in asthma severity by age. [24]

Although Boys had higher statistically significant propensity to acquire bronchial asthma, gender revealed no difference concerning severity. Our findings go in agreement with the study done in UAE [8] as males were significantly more often reporting asthma (17% vs. 14% among females). In another study done between ages 6-14 years old in Qatar, the prevalence of asthma and allergic rhinitis decreased with increasing age. There were statistically significant differences between sexes, males had more asthma, allergic rhinitis, and chest infections compared to females. [15] In other studies the pattern was found to be different where a female-to-male prevalence was at least 50:50. [25]

The studies done in UAE have proved that boys were more prone to get bronchial asthma in comparison with girls.[8,21] Higher exposure of males to outdoor allergens may partially explain these findings because male adolescents tend to spend most of their time outside home, as opposed to their less outgoing and often more culturally oriented female counterparts. Emirian students and those in governmental schools were more affected with bronchial asthma. Again, this was in consistence with Alain study 2009, where UAE nationality children were more affected than other nationalities. [8] In what is believed is, private schools are usually more careful in keeping the maintenance processes of the air conditioning systems and cleaning procedures of the classrooms and school environments, consequently keeping what is known as "Bronchial Asthma Friendly School Environment". Besides, locals usually prefer attaching their children to governmental schools. Some parameters of socio-demographic characteristics were studied in relation to the development of bronchial asthma. Parent's education inconsistently seemed to affect the prevalence of bronchial asthma among their children. Although apparently higher among low educated mothers, illiterate fathers had statistically significant higher percentage of asthmatic children. More than half of the study students had parents with university degrees. This goes in consistence with another study done among children aged 6-7 years in Rome which showed that the prevalence of physician diagnosis of asthma increased as father"s education decreased and the prevalence of severe asthma increased as both maternal and paternal educational levels decreased and lifetime hospitalization for asthma was strongly associated with both parental education.(26)

In parallel again with the case control study which was done in Iraq between years 2000-2002, which gave evidence that a low level of education among parents acted as a significant risk factor for development of asthma. (24) This finding was also supported by many other studies as those done in Brazil, Turkey and Sri Lanka. (27-29) with less educated families, there are adverse environmental factors such as tobacco smoking, crowding, bad nutrition and housing conditions. These factors will make children of less educated mothers and fathers more susceptible to aeroallergen in addition to less medical care. (24) Concerning living conditions, there are doubts that highly likely they can affect the health status of people. Barker et al., (2002) (30) stated that although living conditions in adult life do not seem to be important, the reverse is true regarding children and young adults. In this study crowding index showed no significant association with development of bronchial asthma among the study students. Although non-significant, the prevalence of persistent asthma was higher among those living in houses with 5 persons or more per room in comparison with those living in houses with less than 2 persons and less than five persons per room. A case-control study in Iraq found that the crowding rate of >5 person was a significant risk factor for asthma development. (24) In our study, more than 70% of the study students were found to have homes with low crowding index.

As regards the room ventilation expressed by the number of windows in the room, the prevalence was found to increase with the decrease of number of windows, however this was not significant. In this study no clear relation could be detected between room ventilation and severity of bronchial asthma. These findings can simply be explained by the fact that Dubai is a very hot country during almost all the year with consequent total dependence of the people on air conditioning system. People cannot rely on windows as a source of natural ventilation due to the very hot and humid natural air. On the other hand, a case-control study which included 120 cases of asthmatic children and a doubled number of controls proved that absence of windows in living rooms was among factors associated with presence of symptoms of asthma. (31)

Although family history of asthma; allergies and obesity was not statistically significantly associated with asthma severity it was found that prevalence of asthma was higher among children with family history of bronchial asthma also it was among the factors that expressed a significant effect on developing bronchial asthma among children with around five times risk. A significant risk of developing asthma was elucidated among students with family history of asthma, allergies and obesity. About 19% of the study students, had positive family history of asthma with almost one third of them recorded family history of different types of allergic disorders? This goes in agreement with Alain study (8) as the family history of asthma was the strongest predictor of asthma. Another study in Iraq showed positive association between family history and asthma whether among father, or mother or sibling. (24) Again those finding are in consistent with many other studies elsewhere in the world.(27,32,33) The association between the risk of getting bronchial asthma and family history of obesity can be explained as both conditions caused by shared genetic risk factors.(34)

Conclusion

It was brought out that 16.7% of the study students have had an asthma attack at some point of time with ever complaining of chest wheeze where near three fourths of them complained of this wheeze during the past 12 months prior to the research. Early onset of asthmatic attacks was clearly eminent among the study sample where 67.1% of them had their first attacks before six years old with a mean age of 5.0 ± 2.9 years for onset of the first attacks. Although Boys had higher statistically significant propensity to acquire bronchial asthma, gender revealed no difference concerning severity. Emirian students and those in governmental schools were more affected with bronchial asthma. Although apparently higher among low educated mothers, illiterate fathers had statistically significant higher percentage of asthmatic children.

Recommendations

Develop a national asthma surveillance system for screening bronchial asthma among school children. This could have the advantages of early detection of cases in the pre-symptomatic stage especially at young age. This ensures no asthma cases are overlooked. Reduce socioeconomic disparities in childhood asthma outcomes. 2- Launch a national asthma public education campaign to: Improve asthma awareness among students, their families, school staff and the public. Promote asthma-safe home environments. Promote asthma-friendly schools and school-based asthma programs.

References

1. National Asthma Education and Prevention Program: Expert panel report III: Guidelines for the diagnosis and management of asthma. Bethesda: National Heart, Lung, and Blood Institute 2007. [Cited on January 30, 2011]. Available from: www.nhlbi.nih.gov/guidelines/asthma/asthgdln.htm.
2. Elamin EM. Asthma and obesity: a real connection or a casual association? Chest journal 2004 Jun; 125(6):1972-4.
3. Lai CK, Beasley R, Crane J, Foliaki S, Shah J, Weiland S. Global variation in the prevalence and severity of asthma symptoms: phase three of the International Study of Asthma and Allergies in Childhood (ISAAC). Thorax 2009 Jun; 64(6):476-83.
4. Bisgaard H, Szefler, S. Prevalence of asthma-like symptoms in young children. Pediatr Pulmonol 2007 Aug; 42(8):723-8.
5. Bateman ED, Hurd SS, Barnes PJ, Bousquet J, Drazen JM, FitzGerald MM, Gibson P, Ohta K, O"Byrne P. Pedersen SE, Pizzichini E, Sullivan SD, Wenzel SE, Zar HJ. Global strategy for asthma management and prevention: GINA executive summary. Eur Respir J 2008 Jan; 31(1):143-78.
6. Akinbami L. Asthma prevalence, health care use and mortality: United States 2003-05, CDC National Center for Health Statistics 2006. [Cited on February 5, 2011].

Available from: http://www.cdc.gov/nchs/data/hestat/asthma03-05/asthma03-05.htm

7. DeFrances CJ, Cullen KA, Kozak LJ. National Hospital Discharge Survey: 2005 Annual Summary with Detailed Diagnosis and Procedure Data. National Center for Health Statistics. Vital Health Statistics 13 2007 Dec ;(165):1-209.
8. Alsuwaidi S, Adulle A, Bernsen R. Prevalence and Risk Factors of Asthma among Adolescents and Their Parents in Al-Ain (United Arab Emirates). Respiration 2010; 79(2):105-11.
9. Tarlo SM, Balmes J, Balkissoon R, Beach J, Beckett W, Bernstein D, Blanc PD, Brooks SM, Cowl CT, Daroowalla F, Harber P, Lemiere C, Liss GM, Pacheco KA, Redlich CA, Rowe B, Heitzer J. Diagnosis and management of work-related asthma: American College Of Chest Physicians Consensus Statement. Chest 2008 Sep; 134 (3 Suppl):1S-41S.
10. Data from National Health Review Survey. National Center for Health Statistics. U.S. Department Of Health and Human Services. Center for Disease Control and Prevention 2006. [Cited on 10/12/2010]. Available from: http://www.cdc.gov/asthma/NHIS/06/Data.htm
11. Health 4 Kids. Health Canada 2008. [Cited on January 7, 2011]. Available from: http: www.hc-sc.gc.ca/english/for_you/health4kids/body/asthma.htm.
12. Pearce N, Aït-Khaled N, Beasley R, Mallol J, Keil U, Mitchell E, Robertson C. Worldwide trends in the prevalence of asthma symptoms: phase III of the International Study of Asthma and Allergies in Childhood (ISAAC). Thorax 2007 Sep; 62(9):758-66.
13. American Lung Association, Epidemiology and Statistics Unit, Research and Program Services. Trends in Asthma Morbidity and Mortality 2009. [Cited on January 20, 2011]. Available from: http://www.lungusa.org/finding-cures/our-research/trend-reports/asthma-trendreport. pdf
14. Zedan M, Settin A, Farag M, Ezz-Elregal M, Osman E, Fouda A. Prevalence of bronchial asthma among Egyptian school children, Egyptian Journal of Broncho logy 2009 Dec; 3(2):124-130.

15. Janahi IA, Bener A, Bush A. Prevalence of Asthma among Qatari Schoolchildren: International Study of Asthma and Allergies in Childhood, Qatar, Pediatr Pulmonol 2006 Jan; 41(1):80-6.
16. Harfi H, AlAbbad K, Alsaeed AH. Decreased Prevalence of Allergic Rhinitis, Asthma and Eczema in Riyadh City, Saudi Arabia, Trends in Medical Research 2010;5(2): 57-62.
17. Al-Rename BM, Al-Rawas OA, Al-Riyami AA, Jasim LG, Mohammed AJ. A relatively high prevalence and severity of asthma, allergic rhinitis and atopic eczema in schoolchildren in the Sultanate of Oman. Respirology 2003 Mar; 8(1):69-76.
18. Sears MR, Greene JM, Willan AR, Wiecek EM, Taylor DR, Flannery EM, Cowan JO, Herbison GP, Silva PA, Poulton R. A longitudinal, population-based, cohort study of childhood asthma followed to adulthood. N Engl J Med 2003 Oct 9; 349(15):1414-22.
19. Akinbami LJ. The State of Childhood Asthma, United States, 1980-2005. Adv Data 2006 Dec; 12(381):1-24.
20. Lieu TA, Lozano P, Finkelstein JA, Chi FW, Jensvold NG, Capra AM, Queensberry CP, Selby JV, Farber HJ. Racial/Ethnic Variation in Asthma Status and Management Practices among Children in Managed Medicaid. Pediatrics 2002 May; 109(5):857-65.
21. Bener A, Abdulrazzaq YM, Debuse P, Al-Mutawwa J. Prevalence of asthma among Emirates school children. Eur J Epidemiol 1994 Jun; 10(3):271-8.
22. Al-Maskari F, Bener A, al-Kaabi A, al-Suwaidi N, Norman N, Brebner J. Asthma and respiratory symptoms among school children in United Arab Emirates. Allerg Immunol (Paris) 2000 Apr; 32(4):159-63.
23. Lam DSY, Leung SP, So KT. Age of Onset of Asthma Symptoms. HK J Paediatr (New Series) 2007; 12(1):11-14.
24. Al-Kubaisy W, Ali SH, Al-Thamiri D. Risk factors for asthma among primary school children in Baghdad, Iraq. Saudi Med J 2005 Mar; 26(3):460-6.
25. Almqvist C, Worm M, Leynaert B. Gender: Impact of gender on asthma in childhood and adolescence: a GA2LEN review. Allergy 2008 Jan; 63(1):47-57.

26. Cesarani G, Farchi S, Davoli M, Forastiere F, Perucci CA. Individual and area-based indicators of socioeconomic status and childhood asthma. Eur Respir J 2003 ct; 22(4):619-24.
27. Chatkin MN, Menezes AM, Victora CG, Barros FC. High prevalence of asthma in preschool children in southern Brazil: a population-based study. Pediatr Pulmonol 2003 Apr;35(4):296-301.
28. Ece A, Ceylan A, Saraclar Y, Saka G, Gürkan F, Haspolat K. Prevalence of asthma and other allergic disorders among schoolchildren in Diyarbakir, Turkey. Turk J Pediatr 2001 Oct- Dec; 43(4):286-92.
29. Karunasekera KA, Jayasinghe JA, Alwis LW. Risk factors of childhood asthma: a Sri Lanka study. J Trop Pediatr 2001 Jun; 47(3):142-5.
30. Economist Intelligence Unit Quality of Life Index: UAE ranks number one in Mena, (The Ultimate Middle East Business Resource). [Cited 2011 Feb 29]. Available from: http://www.AMEinf.com
31. Pokharel PK, Bhatta NK, Pandey RM, Erkki K .Asthma symptomatics school children of Sonapur. Kathmandu Univ Med J (KUMJ) 2007 Oct-Dec;5(4):484-7.
32. Liebhart J, Malolepszy J, Wojtyniak B, Pisiewicz K, Plusa T, Gladysz U. Polish Multicentre Study of Epidemiology of Allergic Diseases: Prevalence and risk factors for asthma in Poland: results from the PMSEAD study. J Investig Allergol Clin Immunol 2007; 17(6):367-74.
33. Burke W, Fesinmeyer M, Reed K, Hampson L, Carlsten C. Family history as a predictor of asthma risk. Am J Prev Med 2003 Feb; 24(2):160-9.
34. Hallstrand TS, Fischer ME, Wurfel MM, Afari N, Buchwald D, Goldberg J. Genetic pleiotropy between asthma and obesity in a community-based sample of twins. J Allergy Clin Immunol 2005 Dec; 116(6):1235-41.

Risk factors analysis for childhood asthma in Dubai, UAE

AlBehandy NS,[1] Hussein H,[1] Al Faisal W,[1] El Sawaf E,[2] Wasfy A,[2] Alshareef N,[1] Altheeb AAS,[1]

[1] School and Educational Institutions Health Unit, Health Affars Department, Primary Health Care Services Sector, Dubai Health Authority.

[2] Staff Development, Health Centers Department. Primary Health Care Services Sector, Dubai Health Authority

Key Words: Childhood Asthma, Risk Factors, Dubai

Conflict of interest: The authors declare that they don't have any conflict of interest.

Correspondence to: Dr. Hamid Hussain: hyhussain@dha.gov.ae

Abstract

Background: Asthma is a large and growing threat to children's health and well-being. It affects 5-10% of the population or an estimated 23.4 million persons, including 7 million children in U.S. Asthma is the most common chronic disease of childhood. Almost 1 in 8 school-aged children are affected by asthma, and 10% of children (compared with 5% of adults) take medication for it.**Objectives:** Studying Risk factors for childhood asthma in Dubai, UAE **Methodology: A** cross-sectional study conducted among multistage stratified randomly selected students sample in preparatory and secondary schools "Governmental and Private" in Dubai, U.A.E , The total sample size reached 1639 students.

Results: parental education, crowding index and number of windows per room. It can be noted that as regards father education the highest prevalence of asthma was seen among students whose fathers were of lower education (illiterate 26.7%) as compared to those whose fathers were of university education (15.3%) with the exception of those in preparatory school (14.3%). Students whose fathers were secondary educated had a significant risk of 1.4 times more than those whose fathers were university educated and 2.1 times higher for those whose fathers were illiterate than those whose fathers were university educated . The prevalence of persistent asthma among asthmatic students was higher among the older age groups (31.3%, 26.3% and 53.8% in students of 13-<15, 15-<17 and 17+ years of age respectively) compared to those of <13 years of age (15.9%). A significant elevated risk was found among students in the 13-<15 years of age group

(OR=2.4) and those of 17+ years of age group (OR=6.2). Sex, nationality and type of school revealed no statistical significant relation with severity of asthma. **Conclusion:** There are many risk factors playing significant role in diseases prevalence and diseases severity and clinical presentation, which needs to be well addressed to be able to modified as a part of diseases management protocol .**Recommendations:** Working at risk factor manipulation level through setting up long term preventive and intervention community and family based programs to modify asthma prevalence and clinical presentations.

Introduction

Asthma is a large and growing threat to children's health and well-being.[1] It affects 5-10% of the population or an estimated 23.4 million persons, including 7 million children in the U.S.[2] Asthma is the most common chronic disease of childhood. Almost 1 in 8 school-aged children are affected by asthma, and 10% of children (compared with 5% of adults) take medication for it. [3, 4] Worldwide, an estimated 300 million people are affected by asthma. Based on the application of standardized methods to the measurement of the prevalence of asthma and wheezing illness in children and adults. It appears that the global prevalence of asthma ranges from 1-18% of the population in different countries.[5] There is a good evidence that international differences in asthma symptom prevalence have been reduced, particularly in the 13-14 age group, with decrease in prevalence in North America and Western Europe and increase prevalence in regions where prevalence was previously low. Although there was little change in the overall prevalence of current wheeze, the percentage of children reported to have had asthma increased significantly, possibly reflecting greater awareness of this condition and/or changes in diagnostic practice. The increases in asthma symptoms prevalence in Africa, Latin America and parts of Asia indicate that the global burden of asthma is continuing to rise, but the global prevalence differences are lessening.[6]

Asthma is a leading chronic illness among children and youth in the United States. In 2007, 5.6 million school-aged children and youth (5-17 years old) were reported to currently have asthma; and 2.9 million had an asthma episode or attack within the previous year. On average, in a classroom of 30 children, about 3 are likely to have asthma.

[7]

In a study done in Egypt in 2009 the overall prevalence of asthma among school children was 7.7% (8% in urban areas and 7% in rural areas). [8] In a study conducted in State of Qatar, the school children aged from 6-14 year revealed a prevalence of bronchial asthma as high as 19.8 % in 2004.[9] In between 2007-2009 in Saudi Arabia (Riyadh) , a study among the same age range (6-14) revealed that the prevalence of asthma among school children was 11.4% [10] while in Oman, the prevalence of asthma reached 10.5% and 20.7% in 6-7 and 13-14 years old Omani children respectively. [11]

The World Health Organization (WHO) has estimated that 15 million disability-adjusted life-years are lost annually due to asthma, representing 1% of the total global disease burden. Annual worldwide deaths from asthma have been estimated at 250,000 and mortality does not appear to correlate well with prevalence. There are insufficient data to fully explain the variations in prevalence within and between populations. Although from the perspective of both the patient and society the cost to control asthma seems high, the cost of not treating asthma correctly is even higher.[5] Children with asthma are at an increased risk of experiencing asthma-related respiratory symptoms in adult life.[12] Asthma is one of the leading causes of school absenteeism. In 2003, an estimated 12.8 million school days were missed due to asthma among more than 4 million children who reported at least one asthma attack in the preceding year.[13] Low-income populations, minorities, and children living in inner cities experience more emergency department visits, hospitalizations, and deaths due to asthma than the general population.[14]

Two old studies on 1994 and 2000 in the UAE among students aged 6-13 showed that the prevalence of asthma was 13,6 % [15] and 13 % [16] respectively. In a recent study in the UAE, in Alain area which was held between 2007- 2010 showed that the prevalence of asthma in the group aged 13-19 years was 16%, while that in the adult group 19 years and above was 12%.[17]

Objective

Studying risk factors of childhood asthma in Dubai, UAE.

Methodology

This is a cross sectional study, conducted among students in preparatory and secondary schools "Governmental and Private" in Dubai, U.A.E. Computer program EPI-Info version "6.04" was used for calculation of the minimum sample size required. According to a recent study [17] the prevalence of asthma among adolescent in the UAE was found to be 16%, using 3 % degree of precision, 95% confidence interval and 1.5% design effect, the minimum sample size required was 855. A list of schools was obtained from the knowledge and Human Development Authority. Dubai includes 183 school spread along two large districts, Bur Dubai and Diera. Bur Dubai includes 90 schools, 69 private and 21 governmental, where Diera includes 93 schools, 72 private and 21 governmental. The numbers of students in preparatory and secondary stages are 42819 and 34299 respectively. Around 20289 of them in governmental schools, while 56829 are in private schools. This gives a total of 77118 students in both regions (private and governmental). A multistage stratified random sample was used. The strata were based upon geographical districts(Bur-Dubai and Diera), type of schools (governmental or private),educational grade (7th through 12th) and sex (males and females). The number of the governmental schools was less than that of private schools (42 and 141 respectively). According to the numbers of schools, a proportional allocation technique was used to determine the required sample size. 16 private schools (8 from Bur Dubai and 8 from Diera), with 4 schools of boys and 4 schools of girls for each district were randomly selected. Also, 4 governmental schools (2 from Bur Dubai and 2 from Diera), with one school for each gender from each district, were randomly selected. From each school one class was selected randomly from each educational grade. All the students in the selected classes were invited to participate in the study and all of them agreed to participate (response rate 100%). The total sample size reached 1639 students.

Results

Table (8) shows the parental education, crowding index and number of windows per room. It can be noted that as regards father education the highest prevalence of asthma was seen among students whose fathers were of lower education (illiterate 26.7%) as compared to those whose fathers were of university education (15.3%) with the exception of those in preparatory school (14.3%). Students whose fathers were secondary educated had a significant risk of 1.4 times more than those whose fathers were university educated and 2.1 times higher for those whose fathers were illiterate than those whose fathers were university educated. As for the mother education, it can be noted that with the exception of the illiterate group, the prevalence increased with decreased educational level of the mother however the risk was not significant. Crowding index showed no significant association with asthma. As regards the room ventilation (number of windows in the room), the prevalence was found to increase with the decrease of number of windows however this was not significant.

Characteristic	Total no. (1639)	Non Asthmatic (n=1366)		Asthmatic (n=273)		OR (95%CI)
		No.	%	No.	%	
Father's Educational level						
University	1062	899	84.7	163	15.3	1
Secondary	321	257	80.1	64	19.9	1.4 (1.0-1.9)*
Preparatory	133	114	85.7	19	14.3	0.9 (0.56-1.5)
Primary	78	63	80.8	15	19.2	1.3 (0.72-2.4)
Illiterate	45	33	73.3	12	26.7	2.1 (1.1-4.0)*
Mother's educational level						
University	855	715	83.6	140	16.4	1
Secondary	424	358	84.4	66	15.6	1.0 (0.67-1.3)
Preparatory	127	102	80.3	25	19.7	1.3 (0.77-2.0)
Primary	137	109	79.6	28	20.4	1.3 (0.83-2.1)
Illiterate	96	82	85.4	14	14.6	0.83 (0.48-1.6)
Crowding index (person\room)						
<2	1209	998	82.5	211	17.5	1
2-	412	353	85.7	59	14.3	0.74(0.57-1.1)
5+	18	15	83.3	3	16.7	0.94(0.17-3.4)
No, of windows in room						
No	62	55	88.7	7	11.3	1
>2	307	258	84.0	49	16.0	1.5 (0.63-3.4)
≤ 2	1270	1053	82.9	217	17.1	1.6 (0.72-3.6)

*$P<0.05$

Table (9) presents the prevalence of asthma according to the family history of asthma and obesity in Dubai 2011. The prevalence of asthma was higher among those with family history of asthma (39.5%) as compared to those with no family history (11.2%) and this yielded a significant risk of 5.2 times more among those with family history of asthma. A significant risk of developing asthma can also be noted among those with family history of allergies (1.5 times) and those with family history of obesity (1.8 times).

Family history	Total no. (1639)	Non Asthmatic (n=1366)		Asthmatic (n=273)		OR (95%CI)
		No.	%	No.	%	
Family history of asthma						
No	1325	1176	88.8	149	11.2	1
Yes	314	190	60.5	124	39.5	5.2 (3.9-6.8)*
Family history of allergies						
No	1097	935	85.2	162	14.8	1
Yes	542	431	79.5	111	20.5	1.5 (1.1-1.9)*
Family history of obesity						
No	1293	1101	85.2	192	14.8	1
Yes	346	265	76.6	81	23.4	1.8 (1.3-2.3)*

* *P<0.05*

Table (10) shows the relationship between demographic characteristics of asthmatic students and asthma severity. The prevalence of persistent asthma among asthmatic students was higher among the older age groups (31.3%, 26.3% and 53.8% in students of 13-<15, 15-<17 and 17+ years of age respectively) compared to those of <13 years of age (15.9%). A significant elevated risk was found among students in the 13-<15 years of age group (OR=2.4) and those of 17+ years of age group (OR=6.2). Sex, nationality and type of school revealed no statistical significant relation with severity of asthma.

Characteristic	Total no. (273)	Intermittent (n=200)		Persistent (n=73)		OR (95%CI)
		No.	%	No.	%	
Age						
11-	69	58	84.1	11	15.9	1
13 -	96	66	68.8	30	31.3	2.4 (1.1-5.2)*
15-	95	70	73.7	25	26.3	1.9 (0.86-4.1)
17+	13	6	46.2	7	53.8	6.2 (1.7-21.8)*
Sex						
Female	123	93	75.6	30	24.4	1
Male	150	107	71.3	43	28.7	1.2 (0.72-2.1)
Nationality						
Non-Locals	111	88	79.3	23	20.7	1
Locals	162	112	69.1	50	30.9	1.73 (0.98-3.0)
School Type						
Private	188	137	72.9	51	27.1	1
Governmental	85	63	74.1	22	25.9	0.91 (0.53-1.7)

*$P<0.05$

Table (11) shows the relationship between family and housing characteristics of asthmatic students and the asthma severity in Dubai 2011. No clear pattern of increasing or decreasing risk of persistent asthma were found with either father"s or mother's educational level. There was also no evidence that crowding index was associated with risk of persistent asthma, although the prevalence of persistent asthma among those living in houses with 5 persons or more per room (33.3%) was higher compared to those living in houses with less than 2 persons per room (28.4%) or 2 to less than 5 persons/room (20.3%). The number of windows in the room was also not associated with risk of persistent asthma.

Characteristic	Total no. (273)	Intermittent (n=200)		Persistent (n=73)		OR (95%CI)
		No.	%	No.	%	
Father's Educational level						
University	163	122	74.8	41	25.2	1
Secondary	64	42	65.6	22	34.4	1.6 (0.83-2.9)
Preparatory	19	17	89.5	2	10.5	0.35 (0.8-1.8)
Primary	15	11	73.3	4	26.7	1.1 (0.33-3.6)
Illiterate	12	8	66.7	4	33.3	1.5 (0.43-5.2)
Mother's educational level						
University	140	106	75.7	34	24.3	1
Secondary	66	43	65.2	23	34.8	1.7 (0.89-3.2)
Preparatory	25	19	76.0	6	24.0	0.99 (3.6-2.7)
Primary	28	21	75.0	7	25.0	1.1 (0.41-2.7)
Illiterate	14	11	78.6	3	21.4	0.85 (0.22-3.2)
Crowding index (person\room)						
<2	211	151	71.6	60	28.4	1
2-	59	47	79.7	12	20.3	0.64 (0.32-1.3)
5+	3	2	66.7	1	33.3	1.3 (0.11-14.1)
No, of windows in room						
No	7	7	100.0	0	0.0	1
>2	49	34	69.4	15	30.6	6.7 (0.31-125.6)
≤2	217	159	73.3	58	26.7	5.5 (0.31-97.8)

Figure (2) shows the distribution of asthmatic children according to the severity of asthma, it can be noted that 73.3% showed intermittent asthma, 20.1% were classified as mild persistent asthma and only 6.6% were considered moderate and severe persistent asthma. However due to the small sample size among moderate and severe persistent asthma they were combined to the mild persistent asthma group and thus asthmatic students were classified as with either intermittent or persistent asthma for subsequent analysis.

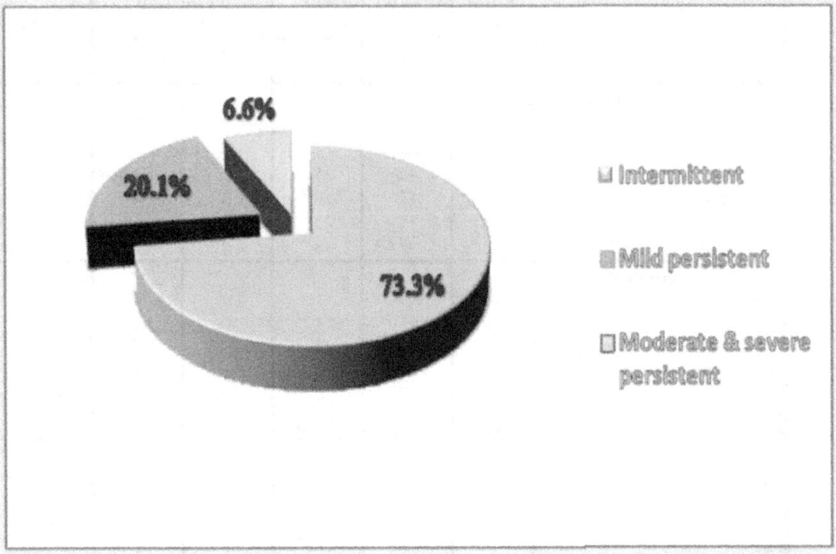

Figure (2): Distribution of asthmatic preparatory and secondary school students according to the severity of asthma

Discussions:

Our study showed that the prevalence of persistent asthma among asthmatic students was higher among the older age groups with a very high significant elevated risk among students aged 17 years and older. This is in contrast with another case control study which was conducted in Baghdad among primary school children aged 6-12 years both showed a decreasing in asthma severity by age.[18] Although Boys had higher statistically significant propensity to acquire bronchial asthma, gender revealed no difference concerning severity. Our findings go in agreement with the study done in the UAE [17] as males were significantly more often reporting asthma (17% vs. 14% among females). In another study done between ages 6-14 years old in Qatar, the prevalence of asthma and allergic rhinitis decreased with increasing age. There were statistically significant differences between sexes, males had more asthma, allergic rhinitis, and chest infections compared to females.[9] In other studies the pattern was found to be different where a female-to-male prevalence was at least 50:50.[19] The studies done in UAE have proved that boys were more prone to get bronchial asthma in comparison with girls. [15,17] Higher exposure of males to outdoor allergens may partially explain these findings because male adolescents tend to spend most of their time outside home, as opposed to their less outgoing and often more culturally oriented female counterparts. Emirian students and those in governmental schools were more affected with bronchial asthma. Again, this was in consistence with Alain study 2009, where UAE nationality children were more affected than other nationalities. [17] In what is believed is, private schools are usually more careful in keeping the maintenance processes of the air conditioning systems and cleaning procedures of the classrooms and school environments, consequently keeping what is known as "Bronchial Asthma Friendly School Environment". Besides, locals usually prefer attaching their children to governmental schools. Some parameters of socio-demographic characteristics were studied in relation to the development of bronchial asthma. Parent's education inconsistently seemed to affect the prevalence of bronchial asthma among their children. Although apparently higher among low educated mothers, illiterate fathers had statistically significant higher percentage of asthmatic children. More than half of the study students had parents with university degrees. This goes in consistence with another study done among children aged 6-7 years in Rome which showed that the prevalence of physician diagnosis of asthma increased as father's education decreased and the prevalence of severe asthma increased as both maternal and paternal educational levels decreased and lifetime hospitalization for asthma was strongly associated with both parental education. [20] In parallel again with the case control study which was done in Iraq between years 2000- 2002, which gave evidence that a low level of education among parents acted as a significant risk factor for development of asthma. [18] This finding was also supported by many other studies as those done in Brazil, Turkey and Sri Lanka.[21-23] With less educated families, there are adverse environmental factors such as tobacco smoking, crowding, bad nutrition and housing conditions. These factors will make children of less educated mothers and fathers more susceptible to aeroallergen in addition to less medical care.[18] Concerning living conditions, there are doubts that highly likely they can affect the health status of people. Barker et al., (2002) [24] stated that although living conditions in adult life do not seem to be important, the reverse is true regarding children and young adults. In this study crowding index showed no significant association with development of bronchial asthma among the study students. Although non-significant, the prevalence of persistent asthma was higher among those living in houses with 5 persons or more per room in comparison with those living in houses with less than 2 persons and less than five persons per room.

A case-control study in Iraq found that the crowding rate of >5 person was a significant risk factor for asthma development. [18] In our study, more than 70% of the study students were found to have homes with low crowding index. As regards the room ventilation expressed by the number of windows in the room, the prevalence was found to increase with the decrease of number of windows, however this was not significant. In this study no clear relation could be detected between room ventilation and severity of bronchial asthma. These findings can simply be explained by the fact that Dubai is a very hot country during almost all the year with consequent total dependence of the people on air conditioning system. People cannot rely on windows as a source of natural ventilation due to the very hot and humid natural air.

On the other hand, a case-control study which included 120 cases of asthmatic children and a doubled number of controls proved that absence of windows in living rooms was among factors associated with presence of symptoms of asthma. [25] Although family history of asthma; allergies and obesity was not statistically significantly associated with asthma severity it was found that prevalence of asthma was higher among children with family history of bronchial asthma also it was among the factors that expressed a significant effect on developing bronchial asthma among children with around five times risk. A significant risk of developing asthma was elucidated among students with family history of asthma, allergies and obesity. About 19% of the study students, had positive family history of asthma with almost one third of them recorded family history of different types of allergic disorders? This goes in agreement with Alain study [17] as the family history of asthma was the strongest predictor of asthma. Another study in Iraq showed positive association between family history and asthma whether among father, or mother or sibling. [18] Again those finding are in consistent with many other studies elsewhere in the world. [21,26,27] The association between the risk of getting bronchial asthma and family history of obesity can be explained as both conditions caused by shared genetic risk factors. [28]

The relation between bronchial asthma and weight of the study students was also investigated. Based on the results of stepwise logistic regression analysis, obesity as an important contributing factor abreast with other factors that were significantly related to the prevalence of asthma namely family history of asthma and being a governmental school student. In this study according to percentile classification, it was shown that, 16% of the study students were overweight while 12.8% were obese. Overweight and obese students were found to have almost doubled risk of developing asthma compared with those who are normal/underweight. Body mass index percentile classification proved that in comparison with normal/underweight students, their overweight and obese male and female counterparts had higher risk of developing bronchial asthma. On the other hand, BMI revealed no relation with severity of asthma in this study. The relationship between body mass index percentiles classification and asthma symptoms among asthmatic students was clear. It can be noted that the percentage of asthmatic students with current wheezing (wheezes in the last 12 months) increased with increasing level of obesity (68.9%, 78% and 82.4% in normal/underweight, overweight and obese students respectively), however it was found to be statistically insignificant. On the other hand, body weight revealed a statistical significant relation with some trends of asthmatic attacks. Those who had more than four attacks of wheeze within the last 12 months were more prevalent among overweight than obese students respectively in comparison to normal weight students were. Same finding was found regards the frequency of asthma symptoms where it was found that the more the weight of the student the more the frequency of asthma attacks, the differences were statistically significant. Sleeping disturbances or speech limitation due to wheezing, and frequency of nocturnal symptoms, wheezing during or after exercise and rate of inhaler use were all apparently higher among obese and overweight asthmatic children.

Conclusion

There are many risk factors playing significant role in diseases prevalence and diseases severity and clinical presentation, which needs to be well addressed to be able to be modified as a part of diseases management protocol

.Recommendation

Working at risk factor manipulation level through setting up long term preventive and intervention community and family based programs to modify asthma prevalence and clinical presentations.

References

1. National Asthma Education and Prevention Program: Expert panel report III: Guidelines for the diagnosis and management of asthma. Bethesda: National Heart, Lung, and Blood Institute 2007. [Cited on January 30, 2011]. Available from: www.nhlbi.nih.gov/guidelines/asthma/asthgdln.htm.
2. Tarlo SM, Balmes J, Balkissoon R, Beach J, Beckett W, Bernstein D, Blanc PD, Brooks SM, Cowl CT, Daroowalla F, Harber P, Lemiere C, Liss GM, Pacheco KA, Redlich CA, Rowe B, Heitzer J. Diagnosis and management of work-related asthma: American College Of Chest Physicians Consensus Statement. Chest 2008 Sep; 134 (3 Suppl):1S-41S.
3. Data from National Health Review Survey. National Center for Health Statistics. U.S. Department Of Health and Human Services. Center for Disease Control and Prevention 2006. [Cited on 10/12/2010]. Available from: http://www.cdc.gov/asthma/NHIS/06/Data.htm
4. Health 4 Kids. Health Canada 2008. [Cited on January 7, 2011]. Available from: http: www.hc-sc.gc.ca/english/for_you/health4kids/body/asthma.htm.
5. Bateman ED, Hurd SS, Barnes PJ, Bousquet J, Drazen JM, FitzGerald MM, Gibson P, Ohta K, O"Byrne P. Pedersen SE, Pizzichini E, Sullivan SD, Wenzel SE, Zar HJ. Global strategy for asthma management and prevention: GINA executive summary. Eur Respir J 2008 Jan; 31(1):143-78.
6. Pearce N, Aït-Khaled N, Beasley R, Mallol J, Keil U, Mitchell E, Robertson C. Worldwide trends in the prevalence of asthma symptoms: phase III of the

International Study of Asthma and Allergies in Childhood (ISAAC). Thorax 2007 Sep; 62(9):758-66.

7. American Lung Association, Epidemiology and Statistics Unit, Research and Program Services. Trends in Asthma Morbidity and Mortality 2009. [Cited on January 20, 2011]. Available from: http://www.lungusa.org/finding-cures/our-research/trend-reports/asthma-trendreport. pdf
8. Zedan M, Settin A, Farag M, Ezz-Elregal M, Osman E, Fouda A. Prevalence of bronchial asthma among Egyptian school children, Egyptian Journal of Broncho logy 2009 Dec; 3(2):124-130.
9. Janahi IA, Bener A, Bush A. Prevalence of Asthma among Qatari Schoolchildren: International Study of Asthma and Allergies in Childhood, Qatar, Pediatr Pulmonol 2006 Jan; 41(1):80-6.
10. Harfi H, AlAbbad K, Alsaeed AH. Decreased Prevalence of Allergic Rhinitis, Asthma and Eczema in Riyadh City, Saudi Arabia, Trends in Medical Research 2010;5(2): 57-62.
11. Al-Riyami BM, Al-Rawas OA, Al-Riyami AA, Jasim LG, Mohammed AJ. A relatively high prevalence and severity of asthma, allergic rhinitis and atopic eczema in schoolchildren in the Sultanate of Oman. Respirology 2003 Mar;8(1):69-76.
12. Sears MR, Greene JM, Willan AR, Wiecek EM, Taylor DR, Flannery EM, Cowan JO, Herbison GP, Silva PA, Poulton R. A longitudinal, population-based, cohort study of childhood asthma followed to adulthood. N Engl J Med 2003 Oct 9; 349(15):1414-22.
13. Akinbami LJ. The State of Childhood Asthma, United States, 1980-2005. Adv Data 2006 Dec; 12(381):1-24.
14. Lieu TA, Lozano P, Finkelstein JA, Chi FW, Jensvold NG, Capra AM, Queensberry CP, Selby JV, Farber HJ. Racial/Ethnic Variation in Asthma Status and Management Practices among Children in Managed Medicaid. Pediatrics 2002 May; 109(5):857-65.
15. Bener A, Abdulrazzaq YM, Debuse P, Al-Mutawwa J. Prevalence of asthma among Emirates school children. Eur J Epidemiol 1994 Jun; 10(3):271-8.

16. Al-Maskari F, Bener A, al-Kaabi A, al-Suwaidi N, Norman N, Brebner J. Asthma and respiratory symptoms among school children in United Arab Emirates. Allerg Immunol (Paris) 2000 Apr; 32(4):159-63.
17. Alsuwaidi S, Adulle A, Bernsen R. Prevalence and Risk Factors of Asthma among Adolescents and Their Parents in Al-Ain (United Arab Emirates). Respiration 2010; 79(2):105-11.
18. Al-Kubaisy W, Ali SH, Al-Thamiri D. Risk factors for asthma among primary school children in Baghdad, Iraq. Saudi Med J 2005 Mar; 26(3):460-6.
19. Almqvist C, Worm M, Leynaert B. Gender: Impact of gender on asthma in childhood and adolescence: a GA2LEN review. Allergy 2008 Jan; 63(1):47-57.
20. Cesaroni G, Farchi S, Davoli M, Forastiere F, Perucci CA. Individual and area-based indicators of socioeconomic status and childhood asthma. Eur Respir J 2003 Oct; 22(4):619-24.
21. Chatkin MN, Menezes AM, Victora CG, Barros FC. High prevalence of asthma in preschool children in southern Brazil: a population-based study. Pediatr Pulmonol 2003 Apr; 35(4):296-301.
22. Ece A, Ceylan A, Saraclar Y, Saka G, Gürkan F, Haspolat K. Prevalence of asthma and other allergic disorders among schoolchildren in Diyarbakir, Turkey. Turk J Pediatr 2001 Oct- Dec; 43(4):286-92.
23. Karunasekera KA, Jayasinghe JA, Alwis LW. Risk factors of childhood asthma: a Sri Lanka study. J Trop Pediatr 2001 Jun; 47(3):142-5.
24. Economist Intelligence Unit Quality of Life Index: UAE ranks number one in Mena, (The Ultimate Middle East Business Resource). [Cited 2011 Feb 29]. Available from: http://www.AMEinf.com
25. Pokharel PK, Bhatta NK, Pandey RM, Erkki K .Asthma symptomatics school children of Sonapur. Kathmandu Univ Med J (KUMJ) 2007 Oct-Dec;5(4):484-7.
26. Liebhart J, Malolepszy J, Wojtyniak B, Pisiewicz K, Plusa T, and Gladysz U. Polish Multicentre Study of Epidemiology of Allergic Diseases: Prevalence and risk factors for asthma in Poland: results from the PMSEAD study. J Investig Allergol Clin Immunol 2007;17(6):367-74.

27. Burke W, Fesinmeyer M, Reed K, Hampson L, Carlsten C. Family history as a predictor of asthma risk. Am J Prev Med 2003 Feb;24(2):160-9.
28. 92. Hallstrand TS, Fischer ME, Wurfel MM, Afari N, Buchwald D, Goldberg J. Genetic pleiotropy between asthma and obesity in a community-based sample of twins. J Allergy Clin Immunol 2005 Dec;116(6):1235-41.

Prevalence of Bronchial Asthma and its association with Obesity and Overweight among Adolescents in Dubai, UAE

AlBehandy NS,[1] Hussein H,[1] Al Faisal W,[1] El Sawaf E,[2] Wasfy A,[2] Alshareef N,[1] Altheeb AAS,[1]

[1] School and Educational Institutions Health Unit, Health Affars Department, Primary Health Care Services Sector, Dubai Health Authority.

[2] Staff Development, Health Centers Department. Primary Health Care Services Sector, Dubai Health Authority

Key Words: Bronchial Asthma, Obesity, Overweight, Dubai Students

Abstract

Background: Globally, epidemiological data estimate that nearly 300 million people worldwide suffer from asthma with expectation that this number will grow by more than 100 million by 2025.**Objectives:** The aim of this study was to gain a better knowledge about the magnitude as well as the association of bronchial asthma with some socio-demographic characteristics, overweight and obesity among preparatory and secondary school students in Dubai. **Methodology:** A cross sectional study was done among students of preparatory and secondary schools (private and governmental schools) in Dubai. Using a stratified random sample technique, the study sample included 1639 children. **Results:** It was brought out that 16.7% of the study students have had an asthma attack at some point of time with ever complaining of chest wheeze where near three fourths of them complained of this wheeze during the past 12 months prior to the research. Emirian students and those in governmental schools were more affected with bronchial asthma. Obesity and overweight expressed as BMI were among factors associated with increase the prevalence of asthma among school students in preparatory and secondary schools abreast with family history of asthma and being male. **Conclusion:** Body weight, family history of bronchial asthma contribute significantly in the development of bronchial asthma. **Recommendations:** Developing a national asthma surveillance system for screening of bronchial asthma among school children, launching a national asthma public education campaigns, targeting childhood overweight and obesity and lunching a prospective study with a large sample size for further investigation of the relation-ship between asthma and Childhood overweight and obesity.

Introduction

Bronchial asthma is defined as a chronic, inflammatory lung disease which characteristically presents by cough, dyspnea, wheezing and chest tightness which occurs in paroxysms and is usually related to specific triggering events involving partial or complete reversible airway narrowing plus increased airways responsiveness to a variety of stimuli.(1) Asthma and obesity are recently evolved into two major public health concerns in developed countries.(2) Asthma prevalence exists globally in wide variations.(3) It is the most common chronic disease facing the childhood in first world countries. Recurrent asthma-like symptoms were reported in proximately 32 percent of preschool children in the United States and Europe.(4) Globally, epidemiologic data estimate that nearly 300 million people worldwide suffer from asthma with expectation that this number will grow by more than 100 million by 2025. Annually 250,000 deaths are attributed to this disease.(5) with approximately 500,000 hospitalizations per year and 13 million missed school days.(6) Asthma is the third-ranking cause of hospitalization among children under 15.(7)
In the UAE, in Alain area a study held between 2007-, 2010 showed that the prevalence of asthma in the study group aged 13–19 years was 16%, while that in the adult group 19 years and above was 12%. (8) On the other hand, obesity showed a marked increase over the last three decades. Childhood obesity has more than tripled in the past 30 years. In United States (U.S), the prevalence of obesity among children aged 6 to 11 years jumped from 6.5% in 1980 to 19.6% in 2008. Among adolescents aged 12 to 19 year, obesity has increased from 5.0% to 18.1% respectively. (9,10) In a study done in United Arab Emirates (UAE) in 2007 on 4381 children aged 5-17 years. The prevalence of overweight and obesity was (21.5% and 13.7%) respectively. More girls than boys were overweight. (11) This parallel increases in the prevalence of obesity and asthma suggests a possible association between both conditions. It has been recognized that obesity is more common among children with asthma. Many studies involving children and adults have observed

associations between asthma and high body mass index BMI. Some studies have shown that with increasing BMI the relative risk of asthma was 2.3 in boys and 1.5 in girls respectively. Obesity is not only a risk factor for the development of asthma, but also it makes current asthma more severe. (12) Children with asthma have a chance of remission from their disease at puberty time. Obesity alters the natural history of the asthma and may prevent this remission; the pathophysiology behind that may be that the inflammatory state of obesity may superimpose that of asthma leading to alteration of natural history of childhood asthma. (13)Most of the reviews show a relation between both asthma and obesity, which are a major public health conditions and threats. Both disorders may share common genetic and environmental causes. There are mechanical, developmental, hormonal, signal transduction, and immunologic reasons for their effects.(14) There seems to be a potential relationship between obesity and early dietary bad habits with bronchial asthma. Obesity may be significantly associated with or be a risk factor of bronchial asthma occurrence and severity

Objectives

To measure the prevalence of bronchial asthma among preparatory and secondary school students in Dubai. To study the association between some socio-demographic characteristics of the study students and bronchial asthma prevalence and severity. To study the association between overweight/ obesity and bronchial asthma prevalence and severity among preparatory and secondary school students in Dubai.

Methodology

a cross sectional study was conducted among the minimum sample size of 855students in preparatory and secondary schools “Governmental and Private” in Dubai, U.A.E.(males and females) Computer program EPI-Info version "6.04” was used for calculation of the minimum sample size required. A list of schools was obtained from the knowledge and Human Development Authority. Dubai includes 183 school spread along two large districts, Bur Dubai and Diera. Bur Dubai includes 90 schools, 69 private and 21 governmental, where Diera includes 93 schools, 72 private and 21 governmental. A multistage stratified random sample was used. The strata were based upon geographical districts (Bur-Dubai and Diera), type of schools (governmental or private), educational grade (7th through 12th) and sex (males and females). The number of the governmental schools was less than that of private schools (42 and 141 respectively). According to the numbers of schools, a proportional allocation technique was used to determine the required sample size. A total of 16 private schools (8 from Bur Dubai and 8 from Diera), with 4 schools of boys and 4 schools of girls for each district were randomly selected. Also, 4 governmental schools (2 from Bur Dubai and 2 from Diera), with one school for each gender from each district, were randomly selected. From each school one class was selected randomly from each educational grade. All the students in the selected classes were invited to participate in the study and all of them agreed to participate (response rate 100%). The total sample size reached 1639 students. The numbers of students in preparatory and secondary stages are 42819 and 34299 respectively. Around 20289 of them in governmental schools, while 56829 are in private schools. This gives a total of 77118 students in both regions (private and governmental). A valid and reliable questionnaire sheet was used to collect data from including , Socio-demographic data, • **Personal data** including age, gender, grade (7th-12th), nationality and schools (governmental and private).• **Family history** of bronchial asthma, obesity and allergy as (allergic rhinitis, eczema, sinusitis, food allergy). Asthma symptoms: 3- Dietary habits: • Adolescent food habits checklist (AFHC) was used to assess dietary habits and behaviors, • Food habit scoring.(104) Pilot test, 3.1.5.2. Physical examination Anthropometric data, height, weight and Body Mass Index. Data were coded and entered into a computer and were analyzed using *SPSS* (version 16). students as well as between students with intermittent and persistent asthma. For all descriptive and analytic statistics, the 5% level was chosen as the level of significance. (109)

Results

Table (9) presents the prevalence of asthma according to the family history of asthma and obesity in Dubai 2011. The prevalence of asthma was higher among those with family history of asthma (39.5%) as compared to those with no family history (11.2%) and this yielded a significant risk of 5.2 times more among those with family history of asthma. A significant risk of developing asthma can also be noted among those with family history of allergies (1.5 times) and those with family history of obesity (1.8 times).

Table (9): Prevalence of asthma among preparatory and secondary school students according to their family history of asthma and obesity (Dubai, 2011)

Family history	Total (1639)	Non Asthmatic (n=1366)		Asthmatic (n=273)		OR (95%CI)
		No.	%	No.	%	
Family history of asthma						
No	1325	1176	88.8	149	11.2	1
Yes	314	190	60.5	124	39.5	5.2 (3.9-6.8)
Family history of allergies						
No	1097	935	85.2	162	14.8	1
Yes	542	431	79.5	111	20.5	1.5 (1.1-1.9)
Family history of obesity						
No	1293	1101	85.2	192	14.8	1
Yes	346	265	76.6	81	23.4	1.8 (1.3-2.3)

-Table (12) shows that by further analysis it was revealed that family history of asthma, allergies and obesity were not statistically significantly associated with asthma severity table.

- Table (13) presents the prevalence of asthma according to the body mass index percentile classification. It can be shown that overweight students have 1.8 times the risk to develop asthma than those who are normal/underweight while obese students have 2.1 times more risk and this was found to be statistically significant

Table (14) presents the prevalence of asthma according to the body mass index percentile classification stratified by sex. Among females those who were overweight had 1.7 times, the risk to develop asthma compared to normal/underweight and this was found to be statistically significant, while those who were obese had 1.1 times the risk but this was not statistically Significant. Among the males, it can be noted that the risk of developing asthma increases with increased level of obesity, it was 1.84 times more among those who were overweight as compared to those who were normal/underweight and 2.4 times more for the obese students and both were found to be statistically significant.

-Table (15) shows the relationship between body mass index percentiles classification and asthma symptoms among asthmatic students. It can be noted that the percentage of asthmatic students with current wheezing (wheezes in the last 12 months) increased with increasing level of obesity (68.1%, 78% and 82.4% in normal/underweight, overweight and obese students respectively), however it was not found to be statistically significant. Studying the number of wheezes attacks within the last 12 months. It can be noted that for each of the different number of attacks categories there was a trend of increase in the percentage of students with the increase in the obesity level, where there were 4-12 attacks among 35.7% obese students compared to, 26.1% among overweight students and 18% among normal/underweight, while there was >12 attacks among 16.7% obese students compared to 6.5% among overweight students and 6.3% among normal students and this increase was found to be statistically significant. The same pattern was also noted in the frequency of asthma symptoms where our analysis showed that daily frequency of asthma symptoms was found among 26.2% obese students compared to 6.5% overweight students and 7.2% normal students while 9.5% of obese students had asthma symptoms over the day compared to 8.7% overweight and 8.1% normal and this was also statistically significant. Sleeping disturbance due to wheezing among asthmatic students with current wheezing was also studied and revealed that as the level of obesity increases there is an increase in the sleeping disturbance percentage among obese students (23.8% for 1 or more/week) compared to overweight (21.7%) and normal students (16.2%) but this was not found to be statistically significant (p=0.407). The same pattern was also noted in the frequency of nocturnal symptoms among students with current wheezing where the percentage also increased with the increase in level of obesity for example 9.5% of obese students had frequent nocturnal symptoms compared to 8.7% overweight students and 4.5% normal students and 14.3% of obese students had this symptom more than 1/week compared to 10.9% overweight and 9.9% normal but the difference was not statistically significant. Studying the speech limitation due to wheezes showed no statistical significant association with body mass index There was also no statistical significant association between wheezing during and after exercise and obesity yet those who suffered from wheezes during or after exercise were more among obese (76.2%) than in overweight (67.4%) and in normal (63.1%). The role of inhalers use was also studied and revealed that for the different categories of inhaler use the more the level of obesity the more the percentage of students where daily inhaler use and use for several times /day among obese students amounted to 14.3 % and 11.9% respectively compared to 8.7% and 6.5% among overweight and 6.3% and 7.2% among normal students however the association was not significant (p=0.672). - Table (16) shows the prevalence of persistent asthma according to the body mass index percentile for age. No clear patterns of risks were observed where the prevalence of persistent asthma among all BMI categories were almost equal (27.8%, 25.4% and 25%).-Table (18) presents the prevalence of asthma according to the AFHC score. The prevalence of asthma was higher among those who had a low AFHC score as compared to those with a high score (17% and 13.5% respectively), the same pattern was seen moong those with medium AFHC score (16.6%) however the risk was not statistically significant. Results were confirmed by considering AFHC score as a continuous variable where when the mean AFHC score among asthmatics (10.6 ± 4.2) was compared with the mean score among non-asthmatics (10.8 ± 4.3) the difference was also found to be non-significant. -Table (19) shows that there was no evidence that the risk of persistent asthma was associated with the AFHC score. The mean AFHC score among intermittent asthmatics (10.8 ± 4.2) was compared with the mean score among persistent asthmatics (10.4 ± 4.4) the difference was also found to be non-significant (t=0.606, p=0.545).

-Table (20) shows the results of stepwise logistic regression analysis for factors related to asthma, which revealed that three factors were significantly related to prevalence of asthma. Family history of asthma was the most significant factor related to prevalence of asthma where students with family history of asthma had 5.4 times the risk in the development of asthma compared to those who had no family history. This was followed by being a male, as it increased the risk of getting asthma to 1.4 followed by the level of obesity where obese students had 2.0 times the risk to develop asthma compared to normal/underweight students, and overweight where the adjusted risk amounted to 1.7 times more than normal/underweight students. Lastly, students in governmental schools were 1.6 times more likely to develop asthma as compared to those in private schools.

Discussions:

Although family history of asthma; allergies and obesity was not statistically significantly associated with asthma severity it was found that prevalence of asthma was higher among children with family history of bronchial asthma also it was among the factors that expressed a significant effect on developing bronchial asthma among children with around five times risk. A significant risk of developing asthma was elucidated among students with family history of asthma, allergies and obesity. About 19% of the study students, had positive family history of asthma with almost one third of them recorded family history of different types of allergic disorders? This goes in agreement with Alain study (8) as the family history of asthma was the strongest predictor of asthma. Another study in Iraq showed positive association between family history and asthma whether among father, or mother or sibling. (111) again those finding are in consistent with many other studies elsewhere in the world. (55,114,119) the association between the risk of getting bronchial asthma and family history of obesity can be explained as both conditions caused by shared genetic risk factors. (92)

The relation between bronchial asthma and weight of the study students was also investigated. Based on the results of stepwise logistic regression analysis, obesity was an important contributing factor abreast with other factors that were significantly related to the prevalence of asthma namely family history of asthma and being a governmental school student. In this study according to percentile classification, it was shown that, 16% of the study students were overweight while 12.8% were obese. Overweight and obese students were found to have almost doubled risk of developing asthma compared with those who are normal/underweight. Body mass index percentile classification proved that in comparison with normal/underweight students, their overweight and obese male and female counterparts had higher risk of developing bronchial asthma. On the other hand, BMI revealed no relation with severity of asthma in this study. The relationship between body mass index percentiles classification and asthma symptoms among asthmatic students was clear. It can be noted that the percentage of asthmatic students with current wheezing (wheezes in the last 12 months) increased with increasing level of obesity (68.9%, 78% and 82.4% in normal/underweight, overweight and obese students respectively), however it was found to be statistically insignificant. On the other hand, body weight revealed a statistical significant relation with some trends of asthmatic attacks. Those who had more than four attacks of wheeze within the last 12 months were more prevalent among overweight than obese students respectively in comparison to normal weight students were. Same finding was found regards the frequency of asthma symptoms where it was found that the more the weight of the student the more the frequency of asthma attacks, the differences were statistically significant. Sleeping disturbances or speech limitation due to wheezing, and frequency of nocturnal symptoms, wheezing during or after exercise and rate of inhaler use were all apparently higher among obese and overweight asthmatic children.

This goes with another study done in Iran, on 903 children, 7 to 11 years of age, through cluster sampling where they applied the International Study of Asthma and Allergies in Childhood (ISAAC) questionnaire. It showed that the prevalence of wheezing among obese and overweight children was 68.75% and 37%, respectively and showed that obese and overweight children had significantly higher prevalence of current wheezing than children of normal weight.(120) Another study was done in Southern California to determine the relation between obesity and new-onset asthma among school children aged 7 to 18 years at time of study entry, through a longitudinal data which examined 3792 participants who were asthma-free at enrollment. New cases of physician-diagnosed asthma, height, weight, lung function, and risk factors for asthma were assessed annually at five school visits between 1993 and 1998. The risk of new onset asthma was higher among children who were overweight. Boys had an increased risk associated with being overweight in comparison with girls. (121)

Again, in Brazil and in 2005 a cross sectional study was done to investigate the relationship between the increases of body mass index and the prevalence and severity of asthma. The study recruited 4010 schoolchildren aged 13 and 14 years. The International Study of Asthma and Allergies in Childhood (ISAAC) phase III was used. Results showed a significant statistical association between the increase in body mass index and the prevalence of wheezing ever, and wheezing with exercise and when stratified by sex, there was a positive association just for wheezing ever for boys and wheezing with exercise for girls. [122] Overall, the relation between obesity/overweight and bronchial asthma has been examined and proved in many studies involving older age groups also. [123-125]

Dietary habits in relation to bronchial asthma were studied. The Adolescent Food Habits Checklist (AFHC) is a tool to measure the healthy eating habits designed specifically for use with adolescents. The AFHC refers to food choice situations in which adolescents are likely to have a degree of personal control. Furthermore, the AFHC focuses specifically on areas of the adolescent diet which present cause for concern, particularly the consumption of energy dense foods and fruit and vegetable intake. Items of this checklist were generated by dietitians and health psychologists. Unsound eating habits contribute to health problems. They tend to be established early in life, and young people who have unhealthy eating habits tend to maintain these habits as they age. [103] it was proved that more than half of the study sample recorded low score AFHC with mean value of 10.8 $\pm$ 4.3, which means bad dietary habits. Although the mean AFHC scores revealed no statistical significant difference in concern with prevalence or severity of asthma but, the prevalence was apparently higher among those who had a low or medium AFHC score as compared to those with a high score however the risk was not statistically significant.

Associations between an unhealthy diet and overweight and the presence of asthma were reported. The high prevalence of childhood asthma in „„western societies"" cannot be explained by genetic background alone and is thus likely to be associated with environment as well as lifestyle. Less physical activity and a dietary change may contribute to the recent increase in asthma and atopy. [126]

There is an evidence that a high level of unsaturated fatty acid dietary intake is related to an increase in prevalence of asthma and chronic obstructive pulmonary disease (COPD). It has been hypothesized that the increase in asthma may, in part, be a consequence of changing diet, and early life dietary exposures might be particularly important in the development of childhood asthma. It is well known that changes in dietary habits, such as increasing salt intake, and decreasing intake of fruit and vegetables, contribute to the rise in asthma and COPD mortality and morbidity. (127) The Mediterranean diet is healthy eating pattern with protective effects on chronic diseases. It represents a set of healthy dietary habits including high consumption of vegetables and fresh fruits, with olive oil as the main source of fat. (128) The effect of this healthy diet was examined in a cross sectional study done in Portugal including 174 asthmatics where it showed that high adherence to Mediterranean diet reduced 78% the risk of non-controlled asthma after adjusting for gender, age, education, inhaled corticosteroids and energy intake. (129) Stepwise logistic regression analysis of the results of this study proved that obesity and overweight expressed as BMI were among the risk factors to increase the prevalence of asthma among preparatory and secondary school students abreast with family history of asthma and being a male student. Also, those in governmental schools were found to have higher risk of developing bronchial asthma in comparison with students in private schools.

Ultimately, bronchial asthma frequently starts in early childhood, but it is very difficult to diagnose in this age group. Symptom history still forms the basis for defining asthma in both clinical and epidemiological settings. Bronchial hyper-responsiveness (BHR) tests only, marginally increased the diagnostic accuracy after symptom history had been taken into account. The diagnosis of childhood asthma should not therefore be overlooked in symptomatic cases with no objective evidence of BHR. Moreover, BHR should not be required for defining asthma in epidemiological studies. (130) as it was stated before, there is a parallel increase in the prevalence of obesity and asthma suggesting an association between both conditions as well as the relative risk of asthma may increase with increased BMI. Moreover, some of the studies in obese asthmatics have tried to find out which disease came first: asthma or obesity. This question remains unclear, but the reciprocal impact of both is evident. Several evident biologic mechanisms exist between asthma and obesity, leading to both direct or indirect association. (131) However, this study considered the impact of overweight and obesity on the prevalence and severity of bronchial asthma.

Conclusions:

Overweight and obese students were found to have almost doubled risk of developing Asthma compared with those who are normal/underweight. Body mass index percentile classification proved that in comparison with normal/underweight students, their overweight and obese male and female counterparts had higher risk of developing bronchial asthma. More than half of the study sample recorded low score AFHC with mean value of 10.8$\pm$4.3. The prevalence of bronchial asthma was apparently higher among those who Targeting childhood obesity and incorporating weight reduction strategies in efforts to reduce the health burden of asthma by decreasing its prevalence and severity and improves the disease control and quality of life in asthmatic patients through: Encouraging physicians and healthcare providers to counsel the following:

i. Dietary Intake:

Limiting consumption of sugar-sweetened beverages and encouraging consumption of diets with recommended quantities of fruits and vegetables.

ii. Physical Activity:

Limiting television and other screen time to 1 or 2 hours per day in children starting as young as age 5 years, and removing television and computer screens from children's primary sleeping area.

iii. Eating Behaviors:

1. Eating breakfast daily.
2. Limiting eating out at restaurants, particularly fast food restaurants.
3. Encouraging family meals in which parents and children eat together.
4. Limiting portion size.

- An advocate for:

i. The federal government to increase physical activity at school through intervention programs, and through creating school environments that support physical activity in general.

ii. Supporting efforts to preserve and enhance parks as areas for physical activity and informing local development initiatives regarding the inclusion of walking and bicycle paths.

- Actively engaging families with parental obesity or maternal diabetes and encouraging an authoritative parenting style in support of increased physical activity and reduced sedentary behavior, providing tangible and motivational support for children.
- Planning communities to encourage physical activity, applying pressure to restaurants and food manufacturers to reduce portion sizes and fat content, restricting access to "junk food" in schools.

- Develop and implement a national agenda for asthma prevention research.

- Consultation to and support of community-based asthma prevention and control programs.

- Partnering with agencies across the emirates to collaborate on asthma initiatives and interventions.

- A prospective study in large sample size to further elucidate:
- The relationship and understand the causal mechanisms of obesity, bad dietary habits and asthma association.
- The virtual causes behind the increased prevalence of bronchial asthma in governmental schools. Had a low or medium AFHC score as compared to those with a high score however, the risk was not statistically significant. □ Stepwise logistic regression analysis of the results of this study proved that obesity and overweight expressed as BMI were among the risk factors to increase the prevalence of asthma among preparatory and secondary school students abreast with family history of asthma and being a male student. In addition, those in governmental schools were found to have higher risk of developing bronchial asthma in comparison with students in private schools.

References

1. National Asthma Education and Prevention Program: Expert panel report III: Guidelines for the diagnosis and management of asthma. Bethesda: National Heart, Lung, and Blood Institute 2007. [Cited on January 30, 2011]. Available from: www.nhlbi.nih.gov/guidelines/asthma/asthgdln.htm.
2. Elamin EM. Asthma and obesity: a real connection or a casual association? Chest journal 2004 Jun; 125(6):1972-4.
3. Lai CK, Beasley R, Crane J, Foliaki S, Shah J, Weiland S. Global variation in the prevalence and severity of asthma symptoms: phase three of the International Study of Asthma and Allergies in Childhood (ISAAC). Thorax 2009 Jun; 64(6):476-83.
4. Bisgaard H, Szefler, S. Prevalence of asthma-like symptoms in young children. Pediatr Pulmonol 2007 Aug; 42(8):723-8.
5. Bateman ED, Hurd SS, Barnes PJ, Bousquet J, Drazen JM, FitzGerald MM, Gibson P, Ohta K, O"Byrne P. Pedersen SE, Pizzichini E, Sullivan SD, Wenzel SE, Zar HJ. Global strategy for asthma management and prevention: GINA executive summary. Eur Respir J 2008 Jan; 31(1):143-78.
6. Akinbami L. Asthma prevalence, health care use and mortality: United States 2003-05, CDC National Center for Health Statistics 2006. [Cited on February 5, 2011]. Available from: http://www.cdc.gov/nchs/data/hestat/asthma03-05/asthma03-05.htm
7. DeFrances CJ, Cullen KA, Kozak LJ. National Hospital Discharge Survey: 2005 Annual Summary with Detailed Diagnosis and Procedure Data. National Center for Health Statistics. Vital Health Statistics 13 2007 Dec ;(165):1-209.
8. Alsowaidi S, Adullc A, Bernsen R. Prevalence and Risk Factors of Asthma among Adolescents and Their Parents in Al-Ain (United Arab Emirates). Respiration 2010; 79(2):105-11.
9. Ogden CL, Carroll MD, Curtin LR, Lamb MM, Flegal KM. Prevalence of high body mass index in US children and adolescents, 2007–2008. JAMA 2010 Jan 20; 303(3):242-9.

10. National Center for Health Statistics. Health, United States, 2004 with Chartbook on Trends in the Health of Americans [pdf 3.8M]. Hyattsville, MD; 2004. [Cited on February 4, 2011]. Available from: http://www.cdc.gov/nchs/data/hus/hus04trend.pdf#070.

11. Malik M, Bakir A. Prevalence of overweight and obesity among children in the United Arab Emirates. Obes Rev 2007 Jan; 8(1):15-20.

12. Moore C. Obesity and Asthma. Report. Business Briefing: US Respiratory Care 2005. [Cited on February 5, 2011]. Available from: http://www.touchrespiratory.com/files/article_pdfs/resp_2265

13. Guerra S, Wright AL, Morgan WJ, Sherrill DL, Holberg CJ, Martinez FD. Persistence of asthma symptoms during adolescence: role of obesity and age of onset of puberty. Am J Resp Crit Care Med 2004 Jul 1; 170(1):78-85.

14. Weiss ST, Shore S. Obesity and Asthma: Direction for research. Am J Resp Crit Care Med 2004 Apr 15; 169(8):963-8.

15. Cowl CT, Daroowalla F, Harber P, Lemiere C, Liss GM, Pacheco KA, Redlich CA, Rowe B,Heitzer J. Diagnosis and management of work-related asthma: American College Of Chest,Physicians Consensus Statement. Chest 2008 Sep; 134 (3 Suppl):1S-41S.

16. Data from National Health Review Survey. National Center for Health Statistics. U.S.Department of Health and Human Services. Center for Disease Control and Prevention 2006. [Cited on 10/12/2010]. Available from: http://www.cdc.gov/asthma/NHIS/06/Data.htm.

17. Health 4 Kids. Health Canada 2008. [Cited on January 7, 2011]. Available from: http: www.hc-sc.gc.ca/english/for_you/health4kids/body/asthma.htm.

18. Pearce N, Aït-Khaled N, Beasley R, Mallol J, Keil U, Mitchell E, Robertson C. Worldwide trends in the prevalence of asthma symptoms: phase III of the International Study of Asthma and Allergies in Childhood (ISAAC). Thorax 2007 Sep;62(9):758-66.

19. American Lung Association, Epidemiology and Statistics Unit, Research and Program Services. Trends in Asthma Morbidity and Mortality 2009. [Cited on January Available from: http://www.lungusa.org/finding-cures/our-research/trend-reports/asthma-trendreport.pdf

20. Zedan M, Settin A, Farag M, Ezz-Elregal M, Osman E, Fouda A. Prevalence of bronchial Asthma among Egyptian schoolchildren, Egyptian Journal of Bronchology 2009 Dec; 3(2):124-130.
21. Janahi IA, Bener A, Bush A. Prevalence of Asthma Among Qatari Schoolchildren: International Study of Asthma and Allergies in Childhood, Qatar, Pediatr Pulmonol 2006 Jan;41(1):80-6.
22. Harfi H, AlAbbad K, Alsaeed AH. Decreased Prevalence of Allergic Rhinitis, Asthma and Eczema in Riyadh City, Saudi Arabia, Trends in Medical Research 2010;5(2): 57-62.
23. Al-Riyami BM, Al-Rawas OA, Al-Riyami AA, Jasim LG, Mohammed AJ. A relatively high prevalence and severity of asthma, allergic rhinitis and atopic eczema in schoolchildren in the Sultanate of Oman. Respirology 2003 Mar; 8(1):69-76.
24. Sears MR, Greene JM, Willan AR, Wiecek EM, Taylor DR, Flannery EM, Cowan JO,Herbison GP, Silva PA, Poulton R. A longitudinal, population-based, cohort study of childhood asthma followed to adulthood. N Engl J Med 2003 Oct 9; 349(15):1414-22.
25. Akinbami LJ. The State of Childhood Asthma, United States, 1980-2005. Adv Data 2006 Dec; 12(381):1-24.
26. Lieu TA, Lozano P, Finkelstein JA, Chi FW, Jensvold NG, Capra AM, Quesenberry CP,Selby JV, Farber HJ. Racial/Ethnic Variation in Asthma Status and Management Practices among Children in Managed Medicaid. Pediatrics 2002 May; 109(5):857-65.
27. Bener A, Abdulrazzaq YM, Debuse P, Al-Mutawwa J. Prevalence of asthma among Emirates school children. Eur J Epidemiol 1994 Jun; 10(3):271-8.
28. Al-Maskari F, Bener A, al-Kaabi A, al-Suwaidi N, Norman N, Brebner J. Asthma and respiratory symptoms among school children in United Arab Emirates. Allerg Immunol (Paris) 2000 Apr;32(4):159-63.
29. Subbarao P, Mandhane P, Sears MR. Asthma: epidemiology, etiology and risk factors.CMAJ 2009 Oct 27;181(9):E181-90.
30. Bateman ED, Boulet LP, Cru AA, FitzGerald M, Haahtela T, Levy ML, O"Byrne P, Ohta K,Paggiaro P, Pedersen SE, Soto-Quiro M, Wong GW, Barnes N, Becker A, Drazen JM, Lemanske RF, Pizichini E, Reddel HK, Sullivan SD, Wenzel S. Global strategy for asthma management And prevention: (update 2010). [Cited on January 30, 2011]. Available from:

http://www.ginasthma.org/pdf/GINA_Report_2010.pdf.
31. Kurukulaaratchy RJ, Fenn MH, Waterhouse LM, Matthews SM, Holgate ST, Arshad SH.Characterization of wheezing phenotypes in the first 10 years of life. Clin Exp Allergy 2003 May; 33(5):573-8
32. Taussig LM, Wright AL, Holberg CJ, Halonen M, Morgan WJ, Martinez FD. Tucson Children's Respiratory Study: 1980 to present. J Allergy Clin Immunol 2003 Apr; 111(4):661-75; quiz 676.
33. De Marco R, Locatelli F, Cerveri I, Bugiani M, Marinoni A, Giammanco G. Incidence and remission of asthma: a retrospective study on the natural history of asthma in Italy. J Allergy Clin Immunol 2002 Aug; 110(2):228-35.
34. Kao CC, See LC, Yan DC, Ou LS, Huang JL. Time trends and seasonal variations in hospital admissions for childhood asthma in Taiwan from 1990 to 1998. Asian Pac J Allergy Immunol 2001 Jun; 19(2):63-8.
35. Smith LA, Hatcher-Ross JL, Wertheimer R, Kahn RS. Rethinking race/ethnicity, income, and childhood asthma: racial/ethnic disparities concentrated among the very poor. Public Health.Rep 2005 Mar-Apr; 120(2):109-16.
36. Akinbami LJ, Schoendorf KC. Trends in childhood asthma: prevalence, health care Utilization and mortality. Pediatrics 2002 Aug; 110(2 Pt 1):315-22.
37. Centers for Disease Control and Prevention. National Center for Health Statistics. Health Data Interactive 2009. [Cited on March 20, 2011]. Available from: http://www.cdc.gov/nchs/hdi.htm.
38. Covar RA, Strunk R, Zeiger RS, Wilson LA, Liu AH, Weiss S, Tonascia J, Spahn JD, Szefler SJ. Predictors of remitting, periodic, and persistent childhood asthma. J Allergy Clin Immunol 2010 Feb; 125(2):359-366.
39. Joshi P, Shaw A, Kakakios A, Isaacs D. Interferon-gamma levels in nasopharyngeal Secretions of infants with respiratory syncytial virus and other respiratory viral infections. Clin Exp Immunol 2003 Jan; 131(1):143-7.
40. Kozyrskyj AL, Ernst P, Becker AB. Increased risk of childhood asthma from antibiotic use in early life. Chest 2007 Jun; 131(6):1753-9.

41. Becker A, Watson W, Ferguson A, Dimich-Ward H, Chan-Yeung M. The Canadian Asthma Primary Prevention Study: outcomes at 2 years of age. J Allergy Clin Immunol 2004 Apr;113(4):650-6.

42. Chan-Yeung M, Ferguson A, Watson W, Dimich-Ward H, Rousseau R, Lilley M, Dybuncio A, Becker A. The Canadian Childhood Asthma Primary Prevention Study: outcomes at 7 years of age. J Allergy Clin Immunol 2005 Jul; 116(1):49-55.

43. Covar RA, Macomber BA, Szefler SJ. Medications as asthma triggers. Immunol Allergy Clin
North Am 2005 Feb; 25(1):169-90.

44. Dell S, To T. Breastfeeding and asthma in young children: findings from a population-based study. Arch Pediatr Adolesc Med 2001 Nov; 155(11):1261-5.

45. Sears MR, Greene JM, Willan AR, Taylor DR, Flannery EM, Cowan JO, Herbison GP,Poulton R. Long-term relation between breastfeeding and development of atopy and asthma in children and young adults: a longitudinal study. Lancet 2002 Sep 21; 360 (9337):901-7.

46. Tattersfield AE, Knox AJ, Britton JR, Hall lp IP. Asthma. Lancet 2002 Oct 26;360(9342):1313-22.

47. Gupta KB, Verma M. Nutrition and Asthma. Lung India 2007; 24(3):105-14.

48. Spivak H, Hewitt MF, Onn A, Half EE. Weight loss and improvement of obesity-related illness in 500 US patients following laparoscopic adjustable gastric banding procedure. Am J Surg 2005 Jan; 189(1):27-32.

49. Sandberg S, Paton JY, Ahola S, McCann DC, McGuinness D, Hillary CR, Oja H. The role of acute and chronic stress in asthma attacks in children. Lancet 2000 Sep 16;356(9234):982-7.

50. Tilles SA. Exercise-induced respiratory symptoms: an epidemic among adolescents. Ann Allergy Asthma Immunol 2010 May; 104(5):361-7.

51. Williams B, Powell A, Hoskins G, Neville R. Exploring and explaining low participation in physical activity among children and young people with asthma: a review. BMC Fam Pract 2008 Jun 30; 9:40.

52. Lucas SR, Platts-Mills TA. Physical activity and exercise in asthma: Relevance to etiology and treatment. J Allergy Clin Immunol 2005 May; 115(5):928-34.

53. Parsons JP, Mastronarde JG. Gastroesophageal reflux disease and asthma. Curr Opin Pulm Med 2010 Jan; 16(1):60-3.

54. Bäcklund AB, Perzanowski MS, Platts-Mills T, Sandström T, Lundbäck B, Rönmark E. Asthma during primary school ages: prevalence, remission and the impact of allergic Sensitization. Allergy 2006 May; 61(5):549-55.

55. Burke W, Fesinmeyer M, Reed K, Hampson L, Carlsten C. Family history as a predictor of Asthma risk. Am J Prev Med 2003 Feb; 24(2):160-9.

56. Schaub B, Lauener R, von Mutius E. The many faces of the hygiene hypothesis. J Allergy Clin Immunol 2006 May; 117(5):969-77.

57. Kinra S, Davey Smith G, Jeffreys M, Gunnell D, Galobardes B, McCarron P. Association between sibship size and allergic diseases in the Glasgow Alumni Study. Thorax 2006 Jan; 61(1):48-53.

58. Goldberg S, Israeli E, Schwartz S, Shochat T, Izbicki G, Toker-Maimon O, Klement E, Picard E. Asthma prevalence, family size, and birth order. Chest 2007 Jun; 131(6):1747-52.

59. Wright RJ, Cohen S, Carey V, Weiss ST, Gold DR. Parental stress as a predictor of wheezing In infancy: a prospective birth-cohort study. Am J Respir Crit Care Med 2002 Feb 1; 165(3):358-65.

60. Klinnert MD, Nelson HS, Price MR, Adinoff AD, Leung DY, Mrazek DA. Onset and persistence of childhood asthma: predictors from infancy. Pediatrics 2001 Oct; 108(4):E69.

61. Asthma 2011. [Cited on May 15, 2011]. Available from : http://www.who.int/mediacentre/factsheets/fs307/en/index.html

62. U.S. Environmental Protection Agency. The Inside Story: A Guide to Indoor Air Quality. November 24, 2009. [Cited on February 1, 2011]. Available from:http://www.epa.gov/iaq/pubs/insidest.html.

63. California Environmental Protection Agency. Proposed Identification of Environmental Tobacco Smoke as a Toxic Air Contaminant. Executive Summary. June 2005.

64. Nielsen KG, Bisgaard H. Hyperventilation with cold versus dry air in 2- to 5-year-old Children with asthma. Am J Respir Crit Care Med 2005 Feb 1; 171(3):238-41.

65. Koskela HO. Cold Air -Provoked Respiratory Symptoms: The Mechanisms and Management. International Journal of Circumpolar Health 2007; 66(2) 91-100.
66. Childhood overweight and obesity WHO 2011. [Cited on January 22, 2011]. Available from: http://www.who.int/dietphysicalactivity/childhood/en/
67. Deurenberg P, Weststrate JA, Seidell JC. Body mass index as a measure of body fatness: age- and sex-specific prediction formulas. Br J Nutr 1991 Mar; 65(2):105-14.
68. Healthy Weight: Assessing Your Weight: BMI: About BMI for Children and Teens".CDC.[Cited on January 6, 2011] Available from: http://www.cdc.gov/healthyweight/assessing/bmi/childrens_bmi/about_childrens_bmi.html.
69. Han JC, Lawlor DA, Kimm SY. Childhood obesity. Lancet 2010 May 15;375(9727):1737-48.
70. Bessesen DH. Update on obesity. J Clin Endocrinol Metab 2008 Jun; 93(6):2027-34.
71. Ahmad QI, Ahmad CB, Ahmad SM. Childhood Obesity. Indian J Endocrinol Metab 2010 Jan-Mar; 14(1): 19–25.
72. The challenge of obesity in the WHO European Region and the strategies for response 2007. [Cited on January 4, 2011]. Available from: http://www.euro.who.int/__data/assets/pdf_file/0010/74746/E90711.pdf
73. Du Toit G, van der Merwe MT. The epidemic of childhood obesity. S Afr Med J 2003 Jan;93(1):49-50.
74. De Onis M, Blossner M. Prevalence and trends of overweight among preschool children in developing countries. Am J Clin Nutr 2000 Oct; 72(4):1032-9.
75. Bener A. Prevalence of obesity, overweight and underweight in Qatari Adolescents. Food Nutr Bull 2006 Mar; 27(1):39-45.
76. El Mouzan MI, Foster PJ, Al Herbish AS, Al Salloum AA, Al Omer AA, Qurachi MM,Kecojevic T. Prevalence of overweight and obesity in Saudi children and adolescents. Ann Saudi Med 2010 May-Jun; 30(3):203-8.
77. Al-haddad FH, Little BB, Abdul Ghafoor AG. Childhood obesity in United Arab Emirates schoolchildren: A national study. Ann Hum Biol 2005 Jan-Feb; 32(1):72-9.

78. Overweight and Obesity. Consequences. Centers for Disease Control and Prevention. 2009. [Cited on December 15, 2010]. Available from: http://www. cdc.gov/NCCDPHP/DNPA/obesity/childhood/consequences.htm

79. Finkelstein EA, Trogdon JG, Cohen JW, Dietz W. Annual medical spending attributable to obesity: Payer- and service-specific estimates. Health Aff (Millwood) 2009 Sep-Oct;28(5):w822-31.

80. U.S. Department of Health and Human Services. The Surgeon General's Call to Action to Prevent and Decrease Overweight and Obesity. Rockville, MD: Public Health Service, Office of the Surgeon General; 2001. [Cited on January 4, 2011]. Available from: http://www.surgeongeneral.gov/topics/obesity/

81. Krebs NF, Jacobson MS. American Academy of Pediatrics. Policy statement. Prevention of pediatric overweight and obesity. Pediatrics 2003 Aug;112(2):424-30.

82. United States Department of Agriculture. MyPyramid: Steps to a Healthier You. 2009. [Cited on January 4, 2011]. Available from: http://www.mypyramid.gov

83. Centers for Disease Control and Prevention. Overweight and Obesity. Contributing Factors 2009. [Cited on February 2, 2011]. Available from: http://www.cdc.gov/NCCDPHP/DNPA/obesity/ childhood/contributing_factors.htm

84. Bellows L, Roach J. Childhood Overweight. Health. Food and Nutrition series. Colorado State University Extension 2010. [Cited on February 5, 2011]. Available from: http://www.ext.colostate.edu/pubs/foodnut/09317.html

85. Faith MS, Scanlon KS, Birch LL, Francis LA, Sherry B. Parent-child feeding strategies and their relationsips to child eating and weight status. Obes Res 2004 Nov;12(11):1711-22.

86. Institute of Medicine. Childhood Obesity in the United States: Facts and Figures. 2004. [Cited on January 4, 2011]. Available from: http://www.iom.edu/Object.File/Master/22/606/FINALfactsandfigures2. Pdf

87. Mannino DM, Mott J, Ferdinands JM, Camargo CA, Friedman M, Greves HM, and Redd SC.Boys with high body masses have an increased risk of developing asthma: findings from the National Longitudinal Survey of Youth (NLSY). Int J Obes (Lond) 2006 Jan; 30(1):6-13.

88. Stenius-Aarniala B, Poussa T, Kvarnström J, Grönlund EL, Ylikahri M, Mustajoki P.

Immediate and long term effects of weight reduction in obese people with asthma: randomized controlled study. BMJ 2000 Mar 25; 320(7238):827-32.

89. El-Baz FM, Abdelaziz EA, Abdelaziz A, Kamel TB, Fahmy A. Impact of obesity and body fat distribution on pulmonary function of Egyptian children. Egy J Bronch 2009; 3 :(1): 49-58.

90. Shore SA. Obesity and asthma: cause for concern. Curr Opin Pharmacol 2006 Jun; 6(3):230-6.

91. Delgado J, Barranco P, Quirce S. Obesity and Asthma. J Investig Allergol Clin Immunol 2008; Vol. 18(6): 420-425.

92. Hallstrand TS, Fischer ME, Wurfel MM, Afari N, Buchwald D, Goldberg J. Genetic pleiotropy between asthma and obesity in a community-based sample of twins. J Allergy Clin Immunol 2005 Dec; 116(6):1235-41.

93. Tantisira KG, Weiss ST. Complex interactions in complex traits: obesity and asthma. Thorax 2001 Sep; 56 Supple 2:ii64-73.

94. Beuther DA, Weiss ST, Sutherland ER. Obesity and asthma. Am J Respir Crit Care Med 2006 Jul 15; 174(2):112-9.

95. Chen Y, Dales R, Jiang Y. The association between obesity nonallergic than allergic adults. Chest 2006 Sep; 130(3):890-5.

96. Weiss ST. Obesity: insight into the origins of asthma. Nat Immunol 2005 Jun; 6(6):537-9.

97. Garcia-Marcos L, Canflanca IM, Garrido JB, Varela AL, Garcia-Hernandez G, Guillen Grima F, Gonzalez-Diaz C, Carvajal-Urueña I, Arnedo-Pena A, Busquets-Monge RM, Morales Suarez-Varela M, Blanco-Quiros A. Relationship of asthma and rhinoconjunctivitis with obesity, exercise and Mediterranean diet in Spanish schoolchildren. Thorax 2007 Jun; 62(6):503-8.

98. Shore SA, Johnston RA. Obesity and asthma. Pharmacol Ther 2006 Apr; 110(1):83-102.

99. Kim JH, Elwood PE, Asher MI. Diet and asthma; looking back, moving forward. Respir Res 2009 Jun 12; 10:49.

100. Peters-Golden M, Swern A, Bird SS, Hustad CM, Grant E, Edelman JM. Influence of body mass index on the response to asthma controller agents. Eur Respir J 2006 Mar; 27(3):495-503.

101. Castro-Rodríguez JA. Relationship between obesity and asthma. Arch Bronconeumol 2007 Mar; 43(3):171-5.

102. Naing L, Winn T, Rusli BN. Practical Issues in Calculating the Sample Size for Prevalence Studies. Medical Statistics 2006; 1:9-14.

103. Asher MI, Keil U, Anderson HR, Beasley R, Crane J, Martinez F, Mitchell EA, Pearce N, Sibbald B, Stewart AW. International study of asthma and allergies in childhood (ISAAC): rationale and methods. Eur Respir J 1995 Mar; 8(3):483-91.

104. Johnson F, Wardle J, Griffith, J. The Adolescent Food Habits Checklist: reliability and validity of a measure of healthy eating behaviour in adolescents. Eur J Clin Nutr 2002 Jul; 56(7):644-9.

105. Centers for Disease Control and Prevention, National Center for Health Statistics. 2000 CDC Growth Charts: United States. [Cited 2011 Jan 21]. Available from: http:// www.cdc.gov/growthcharts/

106. Jelliffe DB, Zefras A, Newman CG. Community nutritional assessment. New York: Oxford University Press 1989; 68-105.

107. World Health Organization. Physical status: The use and interpretation of anthropometry.Report of a WHO Expert Committee. Technical Report Series, No 854. Geneva: WHO; 1995.

108. Cole TJ, Bellizzi MC, Flegal KM, Dietz WH. Establishing a standard definition for child overweight and obesity worldwide: international survey. BMJ 2000 May 6; 320(7244):1240-3.

109. Norman GR, Streiner DL. Biostatistics, the bare essentials, 2nd ed. Hamilton, BC Decker Inc 2000.

110. Lam DSY, Leung SP, So KT. Age of Onset of Asthma Symptoms. HK J Paediatr (New Series) 2007; 12(1):11-14.

111. Al-Kubaisy W, Ali SH, Al-Thamiri D. Risk factors for asthma among primary school children in Baghdad, Iraq. Saudi Med J 2005 Mar; 26(3):460-6.

112. Almqvist C, Worm M, Leynaert B. Gender: Impact of gender on asthma in childhood and adolescence: a GA2LEN review. Allergy 2008 Jan; 63(1):47-57.
113. Cesaroni G, Farchi S, Davoli M, Forastiere F, Perucci CA. Individual and area-based indicators of socioeconomic status and childhood asthma. Eur Respir J 2003 Oct; 22(4):619-24.
114. Chatkin MN, Menezes AM, Victora CG, Barros FC. High prevalence of asthma in Preschool children in southern Brazil: a population-based study. Pediatr Pulmonol 2003 Apr; 35(4):296-301.
115. Ece A, Ceylan A, Saraclar Y, Saka G, Gürkan F, Haspolat K. Prevalence of asthma and other allergic disorders among schoolchildren in Diyarbakir, Turkey. Turk J Pediatr 2001 Oct-Dec; 43(4):286-92.
116. Karunasekera KA, Jayasinghe JA, Alwis LW. Risk factors of childhood asthma: a Sri Lanka study. J Trop Pediatr 2001 Jun; 47(3):142-5.
117. Economist Intelligence Unit Quality of Life Index: UAE ranks number one in Mena, (The Ultimate Middle East Business Resource). [Cited 2011 Feb 29]. Available from: http://www.AMEinf.com
118. Pokharel PK, Bhatta NK, Pandey RM, Erkki K .Asthma symptomatics school children of Sonapur. Kathmandu Univ Med J (KUMJ) 2007 Oct-Dec; 5(4):484-7.
119. Liebhart J, Malolepszy J, Wojtyniak B, Pisiewicz K, Plusa T, and Gladysz U. Polish Multicentre Study of Epidemiology of Allergic Diseases: Prevalence and risk factors for asthma in Poland: results from the PMSEAD study. J Investig Allergol Clin Immunol 2007; 17(6):367-74.
120. Kajbaf TZ, Asar S, Alipoor MR. Relationship between obesity and asthma symptoms among children in Ahvaz, Iran: a cross sectional study. Ital J Pediatr 2011 Jan 6; 37:1.
121. Gilliland FD, Berhane K, Islam T, McConnell R, Gauderman WJ, Gilliland SS, Avol E,Peters JM: Obesity and the risk of newly diagnosed asthma in school-age children. Am J Epidemiol 2003, 158(5):406-15?
122. Cassol VE, Rizzato TM, Teche SP, Basso DF, Hirakata VN, Maldonado M. Prevalence and severity of asthma among adolescents and their relationship with the body mass index. J Pediatr (Rio J) 2005 Jul-Aug; 81(4):305-9.

123. Beuther DA, Sutherland ER. Overweight, obesity, and incident asthma: a meta-analysis of prospective epidemiologic studies. Am J Respir Crit Care Med 2007 Apr 1; 175(7):661-6.
124. Nystad W, Meyer HE, Nafstad P, Tverdal A, Engeland A. Body mass index in relation to adult asthma among 135,000 Norwegian men and women. Am J Epidemiol 2004 Nov 15; 160(10):969-76.
125. Sharma S, Tailor A, Warrington R, Cheang M. Is Obesity Associated with an Increased Risk for Airway Hyper responsiveness and Development of Asthma?. Allergy Asthma Clin Immunol 2008 Jun 15; 4(2):51-8.
126. Bueso AK, Berntsen S, Mowinckel P, Andersen LF, Lødrup Carlsen KC, Carlsen KH. Dietary intake in adolescents with asthma – potential for improvement. Pediatr Allergy Immunol 2011 Feb; 22(1 Pt 1):19-24.
127. Pietrobelli A, De Cristofaro P. Pulmonary health and healthy diet. Allergol et Immunopathology 2008; 36(4):212-4.
128. Schröder H, Marrugat J, Vila J, Covas MI, Elosua R. Adherence to the Traditional Mediterranean Diet Is Inversely Associated with Body Mass Index and Obesity in a Spanish Population. J Nutr 2004 Dec; 134(12):3355-61
129. Barros R, Moreira A, Fonseca J, de Oliveira JF, Delgado L, Castel-Branco MG, Haahtela T, Lopes C, Moreira P. Adherence to the Mediterranean diet and fresh fruit intake are associatedwith improved asthma control. Allergy 2008 Jul; 63(7):917-23.
130. Remes ST, Pekkanen J, Remes K, Salonen RO, Korppi M. In search of childhood asthma: questionnaire, tests of bronchial hyperresponsiveness, and clinical evaluation. Thorax 2002, Feb; 57(2):120-6.
131. Jana Krystofova, Milos Jesenak, Peter Banovcin. Bronchial asthma and obesity in childhood. ACTA MEDICA (Hradec Králové) 2011; 54(3):102–10.

Publisher: Eliva Press Global Ltd

Email: info@elivapress.com

Made in United States
North Haven, CT
04 November 2026

21772731R00065